LASIK
Emergencies

A VIDEO PRIMER

LASIK
Emergencies

A VIDEO PRIMER

Samir A. Melki, MD, PhD

Boston Eye Group and Massachusetts Eye and Ear Infirmary
Department of Ophthalmology
Harvard Medical School
Boston, Massachusetts

Ali Fadlallah, MD, MSc, MPH

Faculty of Medicine
Saint Joseph University
Beirut, Lebanon
Eye and Ear Hospital
Naccache, Lebanon
North American LASIK and Eye Surgery Center
Dubai, United Arab Emirates

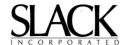

SLACK
INCORPORATED

ISBN: 978-1-63091-262-8

Published by: SLACK Incorporated
                   6900 Grove Road
                   Thorofare, NJ 08086 USA
                   Telephone: 856-848-1000
                   Fax: 856-848-6091
                   www.Healio.com/books

Contact SLACK Incorporated for more information about other books in this field or about the availability of our books from distributors outside the United States.

Library of Congress Cataloging-in-Publication Data

Names: Melki, Samir A., 1965- author. | Fadlallah, Ali, author.
Title: LASIK emergencies : a video primer / Samir A. Melki, Ali Fadlallah.
Description: Thorofare, NJ : Slack Incorporated, [2018] | Includes bibliographical references and index.
Identifiers: LCCN 2017049417| ISBN 9781630912628 (paperback : alk. paper) |
   ISBN 9781630912642 (web) | ISBN 9781630912635 (epub)
Subjects: | MESH: Keratomileusis, Laser In Situ--adverse effects | Intraoperative Complications--etiology | Postoperative Complications--etiology | Surgical Flaps
Classification: LCC RE86 | NLM WW 340 | DDC 617.7/190598--dc23 LC recordavailable at https://lccn.loc.gov/2017049417

For permission to reprint material in another publication, contact SLACK Incorporated. Authorization to photocopy items for internal, personal, or academic use is granted by SLACK Incorporated provided that the appropriate fee is paid directly to Copyright Clearance Center. Prior to photocopying items, please contact the Copyright Clearance Center at 222 Rosewood Drive, Danvers, MA 01923 USA; phone: 978-750-8400; website: www.copyright.com; email: info@copyright.com

Printed in the United States of America.

Last digit is print number: 10 9 8 7 6 5 4 3 2 1

Dedication

To Dr. Dimitri Azar, my refractive surgery mentor, whose deep analysis, honest assessment, and unequalled passion and energy always were and will remain the guiding principles in my daily practice.

To all my fellows who have kept me on my toes and were bold enough to challenge established viewpoints.

To my wife, Rania, and my children, Philip and Alexi, for their love, support, and belief in my work.

—Dr. Samir A. Melki

To all my mentors who guided me day-by-day through all my curriculum.

To my father, Hani, my mother, Maha, my sisters, Laila and Maryam, my wife, Dana, and my daughter, Bella Maha, for their love.

To Abdalla Naqi, for giving me the greatest opportunity a refractive surgeon can receive on his first professional day and for entrusting me with his eyes for LASIK surgery.

—Dr. Ali Fadlallah

Contents

About the Authors

Samir A. Melki, MD, PhD, is the founder and medical director of the Boston Eye Group. He is an attending physician on the Cornea and Refractive Surgery Service at the Massachusetts Eye and Ear Infirmary (Harvard Medical School). Dr. Melki obtained his BSc from the American University of Beirut followed by an MD, PhD degree from Vanderbilt University. He completed his residency at Georgetown University and additional fellowship training at the Massachusetts Eye and Ear Infirmary. Dr. Melki's special interests lie in refractive, corneal, and cataract surgery.

Ali Fadlallah, MD, MSc, MPH, is a fellow of the Harvard Medical School and holds an ophthalmology specialized diploma from Paris-Sorbonne University. He became a European board-certified ophthalmologist after his training in the Hôtel-Dieu de Paris, one of the oldest hospitals in Europe. He holds a medical diploma from Saint Joseph University in Beirut, from where he graduated as a laureate and *magna cum laude.* Dr. Fadlallah is a clinical instructor at Saint Joseph University, Faculty of Medicine, Beirut, Lebanon, and a cornea consultant in affiliated hospitals. He is also an attending LASIK specialist at the North American LASIK Eye Surgery Centre, Dubai, United Arab Emirates.

Preface

The operating room is the worst place to think!

To all of us who operate on a regular basis, encountering complications is an expected fact of life. They can be stressful to both patients and their treating physicians. An unexpected intraoperative event often leads to an adrenaline rush compounded by a sense of impending failure and uncertainty. The chain of events that follows is dictated by how well the surgeon prepared to deal with a particular occurrence, rather than the judgment made in the spur of the moment. The operating room is the least favorable setting for calm and poised decision making. The response to a complication should be based on a previously rehearsed scenario that is automatically implemented as soon as the event occurs. Poor preparation can lead to a rushed, sometimes flawed decision that may result in an undesirable outcome. The rarity of complications in LASIK surgery is a mixed blessing. It is in the extraordinary moment when birds hit an airplane engine that pilot training and preparation become paramount. We hope that this book will allow the beginning as well as the advanced LASIK surgeon to help mentally prepare to turn a complication into a well-managed episode leading to excellent visual recovery.

This video primer is a collection of intraoperative LASIK complications collected over a course of 20 years. Each complication can present with a variety of facets, and we have tried to show as many as possible. The reader is best served by reviewing the videos and the corresponding chapters that list our recommended approach to each of these complications. It has been said that the surgeon who doesn't have complications is the retired surgeon. To all others, anticipation and rigorous preparation is the best way to maneuver through the unexpected and deliver the expected outcome to our patients.

—*Samir A. Melki, MD, PhD*
—*Ali Fadlallah, MD, MSc, MPH*

Foreword

An experienced, meticulous, skillful, and highly respected corneal surgeon shares with the readers of this book his vast refractive surgical experience. Not unlike other top leaders in the field who manage complex surgical procedures and supervise subspecialty fellows, Dr. Samir A. Melki has witnessed his share of unexpected intraoperative events that were managed successfully, transforming every one of these difficult situations into a teaching moment for the reader!

He has done this throughout his career as a prolific author and as a regular speaker at national and international society meetings, sharing his surgical vignettes with other colleagues and with audiences worldwide. Now, he has collaborated with a meticulous and thoughtful coauthor, Dr. Ali Fadlallah, to compile and organize these videos into a series of surgical pearls with unmatched teaching potential for the novice and experienced LASIK surgeon.

Given the rare occurrence of serious complications during LASIK surgery, preoperative preparation is essential for preventing and handling those complications; this video primer will help to minimize rushed or flawed decisions and reduce stress for the patient and treating physician alike.

The major strength of this primer is its ability to provide readers with an accessible means to rehearse scenarios that they may encounter in the operating room and prepare them to handle LASIK complications as soon as they occur.

The educational videos in this book present unique perspectives of LASIK complications. In Chapter 2, for example, several videos of suction loss during femtosecond laser ablation are presented, preparing the reader to handle this complication at various stages of the laser pass. Similarly, the prevention and treatment of epithelial defects are explained in detail in Chapter 7, preparing the reader to properly manage these complications, including the rare occurrence of a defect prior to the laser pass, and to minimize their potential deleterious effects.

I applaud Dr. Melki's and Dr. Fadlallah's efforts in putting together this impressive compendium. The authors have succeeded in achieving the goals of preventing complications, improving intraoperative judgment, and ultimately enhancing the visual outcomes for patients who experience LASIK complications.

—Dimitri Azar, MD, MBA
Senior Director, Verily Life Sciences
Executive Dean and Distinguished Professor
BA Field Chair of Ophthalmological Research
University of Illinois College of Medicine
Chicago, Illinois

1

The Normal LASIK Procedure
A Step-By-Step Surgical Approach

LASIK Steps

Preparing Instruments

LASIK instrument trays can be divided into the following 2 different areas: used instruments area and sterile instruments area.

- Used instruments area
  - Sterile gloves
  - Interface pack (one for each eye)
- Sterile instruments area
  - 2 small piles of 4 × 4 gauze
  - Eye patch (one 4 × 4 gauze folded with tape)
  - Drape: Tegaderm (3M Company; one for each eye or adhesive plastic)
  - 2 balanced salt solution (BSS) tubes per eye
  - 2 packs of Weck-Cel sponges (Beaver Visitec)
  - Syringe filled with BSS (3 cubic centimeters with 25 grams cannula)
  - 2 flap lifters
  - Curved forceps
  - Skin marker

Melki SA, Fadlallah A.
LASIK Emergencies: A Video Primer (pp 1-17).
© 2018 SLACK Incorporated.

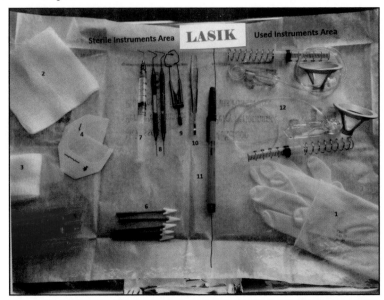

Figure 1-1. LASIK tray: 1-Sterile gloves, 2-4 x 4 gauze, 3-Eye patch, 4-Tegaderm, 5-BSS tubes, 6-Weck-Cel sponges, 7-Syringe filled with BSS, 8-Flap lifters, 9-Eye speculum, 10-Curved forceps, 11-Skin marker, 12-Interface pack.

We advise hanging a photo of the LASIK and photorefractive keratectomy trays in the surgical suite to guide the staff in preparing complete trays (Figure 1-1). This is especially useful in high-volume environments.

Preparing Patient

- Place the head cover (cover hair and ears).
- Place the gauzes between the head cover and the ears (Figures 1-2 and 1-3).
- Apply anesthetic drops (one drop is instilled in each eye).
- Apply Betadine 5% (Alcon Labs) on the patient's skin (mainly on eyebrows, upper eyelid, and lower eyelid).
- Close the contralateral eye.
- Ask the patient to maintain a chin-up position.
  - The patient's hands may rest on his or her chest or he or she may be given a teddy bear to hold and squeeze instead of squeezing his or her eyelids.

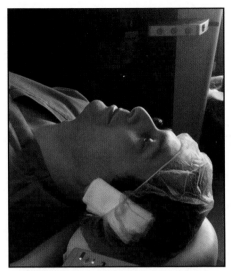

Figure 1-2. Patient should be asked to maintain a chin-up position. The gauze pack in this picture is in the wrong position. The gauze pack should cover the patient's hair and ear to protect him or her from irrigating solutions (see Figure 1-3).

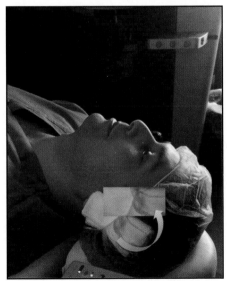

Figure 1-3. Patient in a chin-up position with appropriate gauze position.

Flap Procedure

Femtosecond LASIK

- Preoperative checklist
  - ○ Recheck the patient's name, date of birth, eye being treated, and refractive correction (Table 1-1).
- Explain to the patient that the part of the surgery involving a femtosecond laser will probably be the most uncomfortable for him or her, as he or she may feel pressure and/or black out.
- Initiate the laser platform (Figures 1-4 and 1-5).
  - ○ Enter the patient's name, the patient's date of birth, and the surgeon's name.
  - ○ Choose the procedure: Flap (with the IntraLase [Abbott Medical Optics]).
  - ○ Choose the following flap parameters:
    - Pattern of ablation: Raster cut vs spiral cut (variable; depends on the laser platform and factory recommendation)
    - Hinge position: Usually superior
    - Depth: Between 100 microns (µm) and 110 µm (depends on ablation and residual stromal bed)
    - Flap diameter: Our default preference is 9.1 mm; we prefer a diameter of 8.8 mm in small eyes to avoid air bubbles in the anterior chamber and a minimum of 9.1 mm for hyperopic ablations.
    - Bed energy and spot separation (depends on the laser platform and factory recommendation)
    - Side cuts: Between 60 and 90 degrees (variable; depends on the laser platform and factory recommendation)
    - Side cut energy: Variable (depends on the laser platform and factory recommendation)
    - Pocket
      - ◆ Parameters as set by factory.
      - ◆ ON decreases the risk of opaque bubble layer (OBL).
      - ◆ OFF increases the flap diameter when needed.
      - ◆ Initiate the laser.
  - ○ Verify glass cone integrity (Figures 1-6 and 1-7).

TABLE 1-1

Identification of Sources of Error Specific to Laser Vision Correction*

Error#	Sources of Error Specific to LVC
1	Patient name
2	Date of birth
3	Type of procedure (LASIK, PRK)
4	Aim (distance, near)
5	Optical zone
6	Preoperative sphere: plus or minus
7	Preoperative sphere power: first digit
8	Preoperative sphere: first decimal
9	Preoperative sphere: second decimal
10	Preoperative cylinder power: plus or minus
11	Preoperative cylinder power: first digit
12	Preoperative cylinder power: first decimal
13	Preoperative cylinder power: second decimal
14	Preoperative cylinder axis: first digit
15	Preoperative cylinder axis: second digit
16	Preoperative cylinder axis: third digit
17	Wavescan or laser input sphere: plus or minus
18	Wavescan or laser input sphere: first digit
19	Wavescan or laser input sphere: first decimal
20	Wavescan or laser input sphere: second decimal
21	Wavescan or laser input cylinder power: plus or minus
22	Wavescan or laser input cylinder power: first digit
23	Wavescan or laser input cylinder power: first decimal
24	Wavescan or laser input cylinder power: second decimal
25	Wavescan or laser input cylinder axis: first digit
26	Wavescan or laser input cylinder axis: second digit
27	Wavescan or laser input cylinder axis: third digit
28	Nomogram adjustment

LASIK = laser in situ keratomileusis; LVC = laser vision correction; PRK = photorefractive keratectomy

* This list of 28 items relates to each eye having refractive surgery.

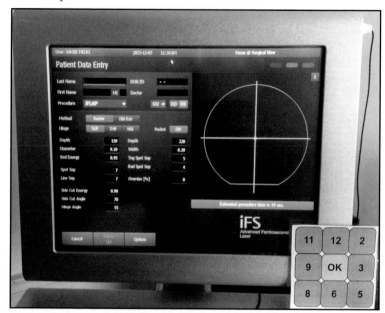

Figure 1-4. IntraLase FS60 (Abbott Medical Optics) platform. Please note the sticker at the bottom right corner of the screen. This has been devised to facilitate communication between the surgeon and the laser operator when indicating in which direction to move a decentered flap. Instead of pointing to the desired direction, the surgeon requests a certain number of clicks in the direction of a certain clock hour.

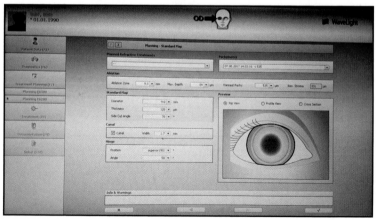

Figure 1-5. WaveLight FS200 (Alcon Labs) platform.

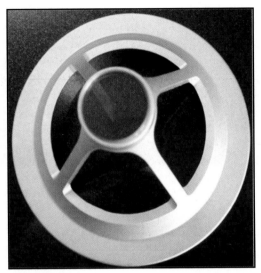

Figure 1-6. IntraLase cone.

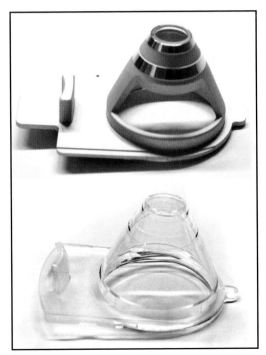

Figure 1-7. WaveLight FS200 cone.

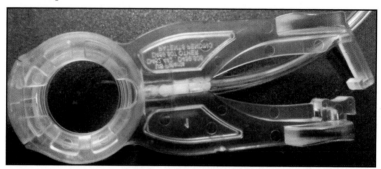

Figure 1-8. IntraLase FS60 suction ring.

- Ensure proper head positioning: Depends mainly on eye and nose configuration.
  - Ask the patient to look in the middle of the rings of lights for the IntraLase platform and toward the green light for the WaveLight FS200 (Alcon Labs).
  - Deep set orbit and large nose: Tilt the patient's head to get access to the cornea and avoid the applanation cone being hindered by the nose bridge.
  - Ask the patient to maintain a chin-up position to optimize eye exposure.
- Applying the suction ring
  - May be done under an excimer or femtosecond laser microscope.
  - With speculum
    - Depends on surgeon preference.
    - Use in case of deep set orbit and excessive eyelids squeezing.
  - Without speculum
    - Depends on surgeon preference.
    - May be helpful sometimes in small palpebral fissure cases.
  - Ring should be decentered to provide 1 mm to 2 mm beyond the superior limbus in the area where the hinge will be made.
    - >2 mm: This may increase the risk of hemorrhage (from limbal vessels) and air bubbles in the anterior chamber.
    - <1 mm: This may induce a decentered flap.
    - IntraLase FS60 (Abbott Medical Optics) suction ring presents marks that can be used for alignment with the pupil (Figure 1-8).
  - After correct ring position is established, apply firm pressure before applying suction.

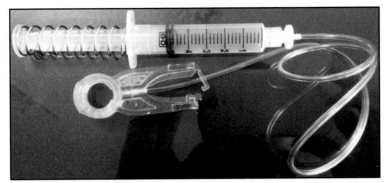

Figure 1-9. Syringe should range between 2 mL and 3 mL (maximum 4 mL) when suction is applied manually.

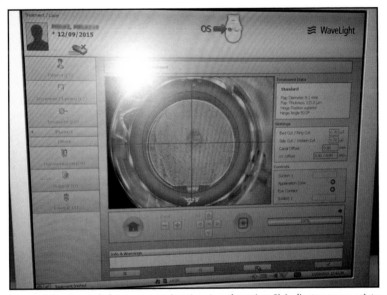

Figure 1-10. Green light on screen (suction 1 and suction 2) indicates appropriate suction pressure.

- ○ Apply suction
  - ▪ Manually for IntraLase platform: Syringe piston should indicate a maximum of 4 mL during suction (Figure 1-9).
  - ▪ Automatically in WaveLight FS200: Accomplished by pressing the suction pedal. Green light on screen indicates appropriate suction pressure (Figure 1-10). Some signs of good suction include mydriasis and blackout.

- Suction may be repeated 3 to 4 times if unsuccessful. Closing the eye for 3 to 4 minutes is needed before any extra attempt (this may decrease chemosis and the risk of extensive subconjunctival hemorrhage). The suction ring can drift due to excessive chemosis. Decentering the suction ring superiorly may facilitate centration while reapplying suction, as the ring tends to slide back into the previously created groove. Consideration can be given to applying a drop of naphazoline to minimize chemosis, but that may lead to pupillary dilation.

- Applying the cone
  - Insert the cone firmly in the femtosecond laser tray without touching the glass (loose cone insertion may end up with difficult docking and a decentered flap).
  - Raise the patient to the glass.
  - Fit the cone in the suction ring.
    - WaveLight FS200
      - The 2 red lights focused on the cornea should cross to be slightly defocused to allow good applanation.
      - Move bed up and laser down to fit the cone inside of the ring. Slight suction ring rotation around the cone may initiate laser activation.
    - IntraLase: 3 different ways are possible
      - Suction ring lock ON: This happens simply by introducing the cone inside of the ring and then releasing the lock (to block cone movement).
      - Suction ring lock OFF: Press on the suction ring when glass touches the upper surface of the ring. Further upper bed movement and laser down movement are needed for applanation.
      - Suction ring lock OFF: Allow 5 to 6 seconds of continuous laser down movement after the glass touches the upper surface of the ring. Then press on the suction ring to allow cone movement inside of the ring. Usually, no further movement is needed for applanation.
  - Hard docking (Figure 1-11)
    - No liquid interface is seen in periphery (between the glass and the cornea).
    - Increases the risk of OBL, but decreases the risk of uncut flap zones.
  - Soft docking (Figure 1-12)

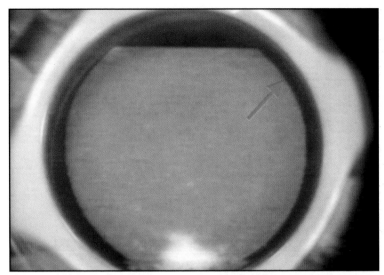

Figure 1-11. Hard docking. No liquid meniscus is seen at glass edges (red arrow).

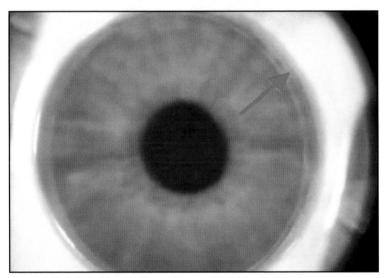

Figure 1-12. Soft docking. Liquid meniscus seen at glass edges (red arrow).

- Liquid interface is seen in the periphery (between the glass and the cornea).
- Decreases the risk of OBL and the risk of air in the anterior chamber, but increases the risk of uncut flap zones (especially on side cut areas).

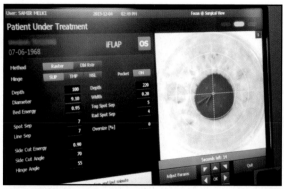

Figure 1-13. Moving the flap outside of the central circle (red arrow) may shrink the flap diameter.

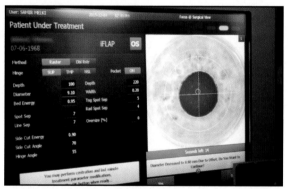

Figure 1-14. Moving the flap outside of the central circle may shrink the flap diameter.

- ○ Look for any contact between the cone and the nose. If there is any, redock with the head now tilted further to the opposite side.
- Flap centering
  - ○ Look on the screen to check how well the cornea is being applanated.
  - ○ Appropriate adjustment on the LASIK flap is done on the laser computer software.
  - ○ Center the flap planned on the computer with the pupil center.
    - With the IntraLase platform, moving the flap outside of the central circle (Figures 1-13 and 1-14) may shrink the flap diameter. Turning the pocket off may help to increase the size of the flap (Figure 1-15).

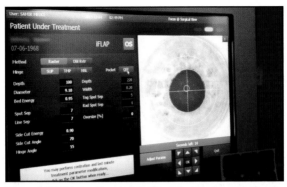

Figure 1-15. Turning the pocket off may help to increase the size of the flap.

- Using a small dial pad (see Figure 1-4) may facilitate communication between the surgeon and the assistant to specify movement directions (eg, to move flap inferiorly, ask assistant to press on arrow corresponding to number 6).
  ○ Apply the laser.
    - 10 seconds to 12 seconds with the IntraLase FS150 (Abbott Medical Optics)
    - 10 seconds to 12 seconds with the WaveLight FS200
    - 20 seconds to 30 seconds with the IntraLase FS60
  ○ Release suction (manually for the IntraLase and by pressing the suction pedal in the WaveLight FS200) and move the laser up.
  ○ Repeat the same procedure on the other eye and move the bed under the excimer laser.
  ○ Remove the speculum if used.

Microkeratome LASIK

- Preoperative checklist
  ○ Recheck the patient's name, date of birth, eye being treated, and refractive correction.
- Explain to the patient that the part of procedure involving a microkeratome will probably be the most uncomfortable for him or her, as he or she may feel pressure and/or black out.
- Head positioning: Depends mainly on eye and nose configuration.
  ○ Deep set orbit and large nose: Tilt the patient's head to get access to the cornea.

- ○ Ask the patient to maintain a chin-up position to optimize eye exposure.
- Instill an anesthetic in the eye.
- Instruct the patient to keep both eyes open.
- Place a plastic drape (Tegaderm) on the upper and lower eyelids.
  - ○ Lashes should be isolated for sterility and to prevent them from jamming the microkeratome.
- Apply speculum on the eye.
  - ○ Maximum exposure is needed to ensure a clear path for the microkeratome.
- Center the eye under the laser by asking the patient to look at the red blinking light (VISX STAR S4 IR [Abbott Medical Optics]) and the green blinking light (WaveLight EX500 [Alcon Labs]).
- Mark the eye inferiorly using a 3 mm marked well: Place 2 to 3 asymmetric marks.
- An anesthetic can be reinstilled.
- Applying the suction ring.
  - ○ Choice of ring depends on factory nomogram (eg, keratometry, pachymetry, ablation zone).
  - ○ Confirm microkeratome readiness prior to suction.
  - ○ Check the microkeratome blade.
  - ○ In deep set orbits, gentle pressure on the speculum may proptose the globe and facilitate suction ring placement.
    - ▪ A chin-up position may be helpful.
  - ○ The suction ring should be centered in a way to provide 1 to 2 mm beyond the superior limbus in the area where the hinge will be made.
    - ▪ > 2 mm: This may increase the risk of hemorrhage.
    - ▪ < 1 mm: This may induce a decentered flap.
  - ○ After establishing the correct ring position, apply firm pressure before applying suction.
  - ○ Apply suction.
    - ▪ Signs of good suction include mydriasis and blackout.
    - ▪ Check intraocular pressure (fixed tonometer or pneumotonometer).
    - ▪ Fix any decentration, buy releasing suction and restarting the procedure.
- Applying the keratome

- The head is dropped on the pivot prior to engagement.
- Look for any contact between the head and the eyelids.
- In cases of a prominent lower cheek, the surgeon may use his or her finger or may ask an assistant to retract the skin.
- The head is activated by pressing the forward pedal.
- After complete rotation, press the backward pedal.
- Release suction.
- If the head stops prematurely, an attempt at continued forward is accepted. Never go backward and then forward. Best practice is to go forward and abort the procedure.
- Release suction.

Excimer Procedure

- Reinstill the anesthetic in the eye.
- Instruct the patient to keep both eyes open.
- Place plastic drape (Tegaderm) on the upper eyelids (for microkeratome LASIK use the same drape).
- Center the eye under the laser by asking the patient to look at the red blinking light (VISX STAR S4 IR) and green blinking light (WaveLight EX500).
- Mark the eye inferiorly using the marking pen; a small marking between the flap and the peripheral cornea is enough for guiding flap repositioning in the femtosecond laser. This step is not needed in microkeratome LASIK.
- An anesthetic can be reinstilled at this step.
- Rinse the surface of the eye with one BSS tube.
- Dry the surface of the eye with a Weck-Cel sponge.
- Lift the flap.
  - Step 1: The flap lifter is introduced perpendicularly at the flap/stroma intersection. The flap interface is penetrated.
  - Step 2: Release the first adherence between the flap and the stroma at the hinge area and then exit at the side cut on the opposite side.
  - Step 3: Flap/stroma adherence is then released by 3 consecutive wiping movements from the hinge toward the inferior flap area. The third wipe movement happens by overlapping at the exit created during step 2.
  - Flap lifting is more simple in microkeratome LASIK because adherence is inexistent.

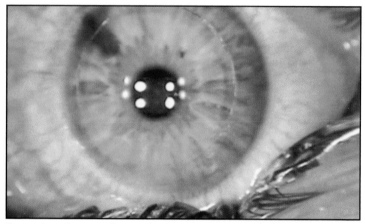

Figure 1-16. Drying with a Weck-Cel sponge between the flap and the cornea gives a symmetrical "ring of light."

- Dry the bed in case of excessive fluid at the stroma interface.
- Measure bed pachymetry (ultrasound measure for VISX STAR S4 IR and optical biometry for WaveLight EX500).
- Tracking is activated (difficult tracking is discussed in upcoming chapters).
  - ∘ Tracking for WaveLight EX500: Foot pedal activation.
  - ∘ Tracking for VISX STAR S4 IR: Manual activation.
- Align reticules with eye marking in case of astigmatism correction to avoid errors induced by cyclotorsion.
- Take a side view to ensure appropriate centration.
- Center the laser treatment on the pupil center.
- Press the laser pedal to activate the excimer laser treatment.
- Holding the head and giving timing update may reassure the patient.
- Irrigate the flap interface with BSS and replace the flap (using 25 grams cannula).
- Irrigate the eye surface with one BSS tube to remove all debris.
- Irrigate the flap interface a second time with BSS using 25 grams cannula and apply some firm pressure on the flap to expel excessive water from under the flap.
- Use a Weck-Cel sponge to dry the intersection between the flap and the cornea to get a symmetrical "ring of light" (Figure 1-16).
  - ∘ Asymmetric "ring of light" is an indirect sign of flap tilt. Flap refloating is warranted to avoid flap striae.

- Instill one antibiotic drop and one steroid drop on the surface of the flap.
- Prepare for the next eye.
- Placing contact lenses or eye shields is not mandatory.

SUGGESTED READING

Carr JD, Stulting RD, Thompson KP, Waring GO III. Laser in situ keratomileusis: surgical technique. *Ophthalmol Clin North Am.* 2001 Jun;14(2):285-94.

Maldonado MJ, Nieto JC, Piñero DP. Advances in technologies for laser-assisted in situ keratomileusis (LASIK) surgery. *Expert Rev Med Devices.* 2008 Mar;5(2):209-29.

Robert, MC, Choi, CJ, Shapiro FE, Urman RD, Melki S. Avoidance of serious medical errors in refractive surgery using a custom preoperative checklist. *J Cataract Refract Surg.* 2015 Oct;41(10):2171-8.

Please see videos on the accompanying website at

www.healio.com/books/lasikvideos

2

Loss of Suction

Etiology and Incidence of Loss of Suction

Loss of suction can occur during flap creation, either with a femtosecond laser or with a microkeratome.[1] Loss of suction can be due to the following:

- Inadequate initial suction
- Patient movement, eye rotation, and/or head tilt
- Flat corneas with dioptric readings of less than 42 diopters (D)
- Smaller palpebral fissure
- Deep set eyes
- Incarcerated conjunctiva

With femtosecond laser, reported loss of suction incidence varies between 0.3% (IntraLase [Abbott Medical Optics]) and 4.4% (VisuMax [Carl Zeiss Meditec Inc]). With microkeratome, loss of suction incidence varies between 0.3% (Amadeus [Abbott Medical Optics]) and 1.2% (Chiron Corneal Shaper [Chiron Vision]).[2,3]

Melki SA, Fadlallah A.
LASIK Emergencies: A Video Primer (pp 19-28).
© 2018 SLACK Incorporated.

Femtosecond LASIK Complications and Immediate Solutions

Complication #1: Loss of Suction (During Raster Cut)

Video section: 1 minute 20 seconds

Platform: IntraLase FS60 kilohertz (kHz) (Abbott Medical Optics)

Flap diameter: 9.3 mm

Flap target depth: 100 microns (μm)

The initial surgery on the right eye resulted in an incomplete flap construction due to suction loss occurring at two-thirds the distance across the planned cut (video 2; time: 1 minute 20 seconds; Figures 2-1 and 2-2).

Some practical measures are as follows:

- Lift up your foot from the laser pedal immediately. This is important to avoid cutting the rest of the flap at a different depth.
- Press "Cancel" on the IntraLase platform or the equivalent on other platforms.
- Do not change the applanation cone to ensure that the repeat cut is at the same depth.
- You may consider changing the suction ring after 2 to 3 unsuccessful attempts.
- Femtosecond laser cut may be repeated.
- The vertical limbal pocket typically created to absorb the cavitation bubbles should be deactivated if already created during the first pass.
- Once a new successful flap is created, start the mechanical flap dissection from the section of the flap that has had one raster pass (ie, the most distal portion from the hinge). This will avoid the possibility of dissecting an area where 2 dissection planes could be present.

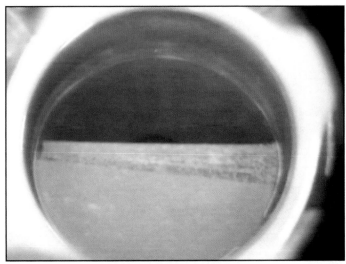

Figure 2-1. Initial surgery resulted in an incomplete flap construction due to suction loss occurring at two-thirds the distance across the planned cut.

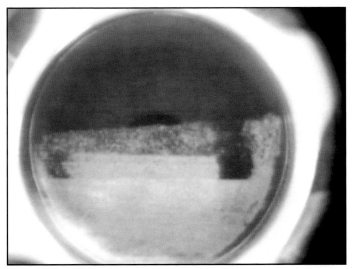

Figure 2-2. Suction ring was reapplied, and the raster pass resulted in complete flap creation. Ablation was subsequently performed on both eyes. Intraoperative corneal pachymetry revealed a flap thickness of 87 μm. On the first day after surgery, the patient had an uncorrected distance visual acuity of 20/25 in each eye, with LASIK flaps clear and well-centered on slit lamp examination. At the 2-month follow-up visit, uncorrected distance visual acuity was 20/20 in each eye.

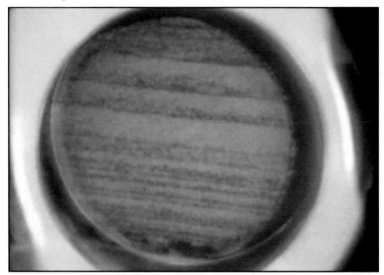

Figure 2-3. Initial surgery resulted in an incomplete flap construction due to suction loss occurring after the raster cut and before the side cut.

Complication #2: Loss of Suction (After Raster Cut, Before or During Side Cut)

When this complication occurs, the flap bed is fully created, but the suction is lost prior to the creation of the side cut. This prevents the flap from being lifted.

Video section: 4 minutes 32 seconds

Platform: IntraLase FS60 kHz

Flap diameter: 9.3 mm

Flap target depth: 100 μm

The initial surgery on the right eye resulted in an incomplete flap construction due to suction loss occurring after the raster cut and before the side cut (video 2; time: 4 minutes 32 seconds; Figures 2-3 and 2-4).

Some practical measures are as follows:

- Lift up your foot from the laser pedal immediately. This is important to avoid cutting the rest of the flap at a different depth.
- The same applanation cone should be used to ensure the same depth of treatment.
- The vertical limbal pocket and the raster cut should be deactivated when attempting a new pass.

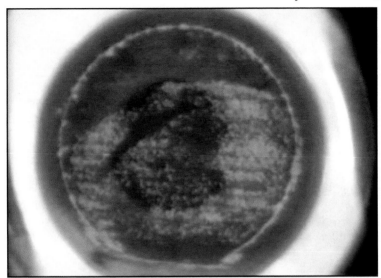

Figure 2-4. Second laser pass was done with disabling the raster cut and decreasing the side cut diameter to 8.7 mm. Ablation was subsequently performed on both eyes. Intraoperative corneal pachymetry revealed a flap thickness of 101 μm. On the first day after surgery, the patient had an uncorrected distance visual acuity of 20/20 in each eye, with LASIK flaps clear and well-centered on slit lamp examination. At the 2-month follow-up visit, uncorrected distance visual acuity was 20/20 in each eye.

- The subsequent side cut should be created within the already-created flap. The laser manufacturers recommend shrinking the subsequent side cut by 0.5 mm. The transient opaque bubble layer pattern remains visible if the suction ring is immediately reapplied, allowing for the identification of the border of the first raster pass.
- If you are unable to set the laser to a "side cut only" pattern, it is okay to repeat the whole treatment while turning off the pocket.

General Practical Measures in Femtosecond LASIK Surgery

Once suction loss is detected, the following measures should be taken:
- Discontinue the laser treatment immediately. Failure to do so may lead to the raster ablation being performed at different depths.
- If suction loss is detected during the raster stage prior to the creation of the side cut, the femtosecond laser cut may be repeated.

- The same applanation cone should be used to ensure the same depth of treatment.
- The suction ring may be exchanged if the surgeon suspects a manufacturing defect.
- The vertical limbal pocket typically created to absorb the cavitation bubbles may be deactivated if already created during the first pass.
- Start the mechanical flap dissection from the section of the flap that has had one raster pass (ie, the most distal portion from the hinge).
- Blunt dissection may result in irregular disrupted flap. Go slower than usual.
- If the loss of suction occurs while creating the side cut, the surgeon must ensure that the subsequent side cut is created within the already-created flap. As stated previously, the laser manufacturers recommend shrinking the subsequent side cut by 0.5 mm. The transient opaque bubble layer pattern remains visible if the suction ring is immediately reapplied, allowing for the identification of the border of the first raster pass.
- If repeated suction attempts prove unsuccessful or results in an irregular flap, surface ablation should be considered over the incomplete flap. This can be performed as early as 1 week after the aborted procedure with the application of mitomycin-C to avoid scarring.

Multiple vacuum applications may not be permissible in certain situations (eg, in patients with glaucoma). There is no evidence of an adverse effect on the retina due to repeated suction application to the globe.

A repeat cut may not be as safe with fast lasers in case the ablation was not immediately interrupted after the loss of suction. A loss of suction in the visual axis with lasers such as the WaveLight FS200 (Alcon Labs) and the IntraLase FS (Abbott Medical Optics) may be best aborted and converted to a future surface ablation. Faster lasers such as these may have cut at a shallower depth prior to laser interruption by the surgeon.

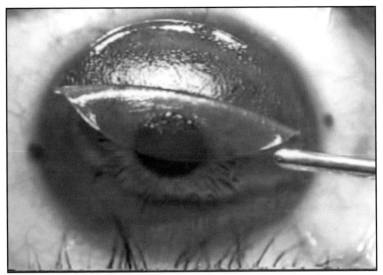

Figure 2-5. Initial surgery resulted in an incomplete flap construction due to suction loss occurring at one-third the distance across the planned cut. Surgery was aborted, and surface refractive procedure was planned 1 week later.

MICROKERATOME LASIK COMPLICATIONS AND IMMEDIATE SOLUTIONS

Complication #3: Loss of Suction During Microkeratome Pass

Video section: 6 minutes 26 seconds

Platform: Hansatome (Bausch + Lomb)

Flap diameter: 9.5 mm

Flap target depth: 120 µm

The initial surgery resulted in an incomplete flap construction due to suction loss occurring at one-third the distance across the planned cut (Figure 2-5).

The following are some practical measures:

- Abort the surgery.
- Assess the exposed stromal surface for excimer laser treatment.
- Plan for a future surface refractive procedure if the extent of the stromal bed created is not adequate to apply the excimer laser treatment.

General Practical Measures in Microkeratome LASIK Surgery

Once suction loss is detected, the following measures should be taken:

- If suction break occurs before any pass, the suction ring may be reapplied.
- Abort the surgery if suction break or jamming occurs during microkeratome pass.
- Assess the available stromal surface for excimer laser treatment.
- Plan for a future surface refractive procedure if the extent of the stromal bed created is not adequate to apply the excimer laser treatment.
- If the suction loss occurs beyond the visual access, treatment can be applied if the stromal bed is adequate for at least 6 mm optical zone treatment. A 5.5 mm optical zone may be considered in spherical treatments less than 3 D in magnitude.
- Avoid manually extending the dissection with a blade.
- When the laser ablation is performed, the flap should be protected from laser exposure, especially in hyperopic treatments.
- If suction loss results in an irregular flap, surface ablation should be considered over the incomplete flap. The timing of the repeat procedure depends on how quickly the surface epithelium is healed. As with femtosecond LASIK surgery, this should be performed with the application of mitomycin-C to avoid scarring.

PREVENTION OF LOSS OF SUCTION

Femtosecond LASIK

The first sign of suction loss is an asymmetric tear meniscus leading to a partial or full loss of applanation. Careful observation during docking of the patient interface and reposition if necessary can be helpful. Additionally, recognizing preoperative risk factors, such as a deep set orbit, and planning accordingly can also be useful in preventing suction loss. Patients who forcefully squeeze their lids may benefit from additional sedation or the placement of a wire lid speculum.

Microkeratome LASIK

As stated above, recognizing preoperative risk factors (eg, a deep set orbit) and planning accordingly may also aid in preventing suction loss. As with femtosecond LASIK, additional sedation or the placement of a wire lid speculum may be useful in patients who forcefully squeeze their lids. The incidence of suction loss may be reduced if the surgeon pays attention to the following guidelines:

- Avoid cutting the flap if the intraocular pressure is low.
- Use larger suction rings in flat corneas.
- Inspect the microkeratome blade under the operating microscope before engaging it in the suction ring to rule out manufacturing or other preoperative damage.

If a case is aborted, we do not recommend switching to surface ablation in the same setting. It may be best to reconsent the patient and proceed with surface ablation on a different day.

REFERENCES

1. Muñoz G, Albarrán-Diego C, Ferrer-Blasco T, Javaloy J, García-Lázaro S. Single versus double femtosecond laser pass for incomplete laser in situ keratomileusis flap in contralateral eyes: visual and optical outcomes. *J Cataract Refract Surg.* 2012;38(1):8-15.
2. Rosman M, Hall RC, Chan C, et al. Comparison of efficacy and safety of laser in situ keratomileusis using 2 femtosecond laser platforms in contralateral eyes. *J Cataract Refract Surg.* 2013;39(7):1066-1073.
3. Ang M, Mehta JS, Rosman M, et al. Visual outcomes comparison of 2 femtosecond laser platforms for laser in situ keratomileusis. *J Cataract Refract Surg.* 2013;39(11):1647-1652.

SUGGESTED READING

Faktorovich E. *Femtodynamics.* Thorofare, NJ: SLACK Inc; 2009.

Melki S, Azar DT. LASIK complications: etiology, management, and prevention. *Surv Ophthalmol.* 2001;46(2):95-116.

Shah DN, Melki SA. Complications of femtosecond-assisted laser in-situ keratomileusis flaps. *Semin Ophthalmol.* 2014;29(5-6):363-375.

Syed ZA, Melki SA. Successful femtosecond LASIK flap creation despite multiple suction losses. *Digit J Ophthalmol.* 2014;20(1):7-9.

Please see videos on the accompanying website at

www.healio.com/books/lasikvideos

3

Air Bubbles in the Anterior Chamber

ETIOLOGY AND INCIDENCE OF AIR BUBBLES IN ANTERIOR CHAMBER

Anterior chamber (AC) gas bubbles are an occurrence specific to the femtosecond laser.[1] It is hypothesized that gas bubbles enter through Schlemm's canal.[2] Some authors believe that the bubbles may be due to misdirected femtosecond laser pulses on the aqueous[3]; however, imaging with optical coherence tomography was performed and does not appear to support the theory that gas bubbles migrate into the AC through the trabecular meshwork.[3] This is not consistent with our experience, where gas bubbles invariably enter the AC through the trabecular meshwork.

Studies comparing complication rates between the microkeratome and femtosecond-created flaps found that gas bubbles were present in the AC only in the femtosecond group (0.3%).[4,5] Air bubbles appear more frequently in the inferonasal quadrant (>50%).[6] When air bubbles are present, they will interfere with pupil tracking in 50% of cases.[6] Surgery can be completed later the same day in almost all cases without further complication by allowing the bubble(s) to resorb.

Melki SA, Fadlallah A.
LASIK Emergencies: A Video Primer (pp 29-37).
© 2018 SLACK Incorporated.

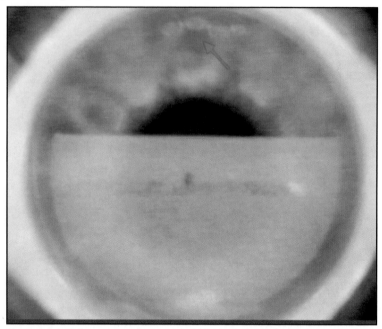

Figure 3-1. Initial surgery resulted in air bubbles in the AC (red arrow).

FEMTOSECOND LASIK COMPLICATIONS AND IMMEDIATE SOLUTIONS

Complication #1: Air Bubbles in Anterior Chamber Not Interfering With Excimer Laser Treatment

Video section: 2 minutes 9 seconds

Platform: IntraLase FS60 kilohertz (kHz) (Abbott Medical Optics)

Flap diameter: 9.3 mm

Flap target depth: 100 microns (μm)

The initial surgery resulted in air bubbles in the AC (video 2; time: 2 minutes 9 seconds; Figures 3-1, 3-2, 3-3, and 3-4).

Some practical measures are as follows:

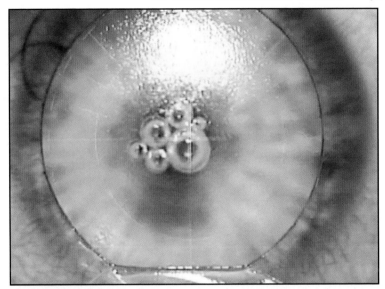

Figure 3-2. VISX brand laser was used for the excimer procedure.

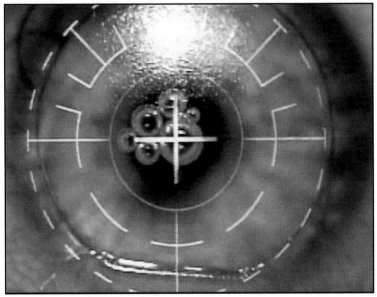

Figure 3-3. Dimming the light during the tracker registration was helpful to activate the tracker.

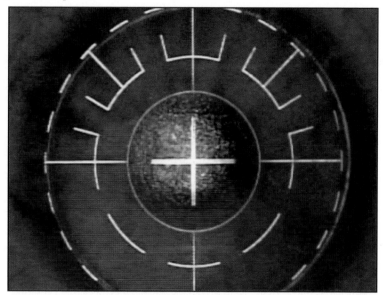

Figure 3-4. Ablation was subsequently performed. On the left eye, the flap diameter was decreased to 8.9 mm. No air bubble was seen in the AC, and the excimer procedure was uneventful. On the first day after surgery, the patient had an uncorrected distance visual acuity of 20/25 in each eye with LASIK flaps clear and well-centered on slit lamp examination. At his 2-month follow-up visit, uncorrected distance visual acuity was 20/20 in each eye.

- Decrease flap diameter on the fellow eye by 0.5 mm and turn off the pocket.
- During excimer laser treatment, dimming the light during the tracker registration can be helpful to allow more reliable pupil tracking.

Complication #2: Air Bubbles in Anterior Chamber Interfering With Excimer Laser Treatment

Video section: 3 minutes 48 seconds
Platform: Wavelight FS200 (Alcon Labs)
Flap diameter: 9.3 mm
Flap target depth: 100 μm

The initial surgery resulted in air bubbles in the AC (video 2; time: 3 minutes 48 seconds; Figures 3-5, 3-6, 3-7, 3-8, and 3-9).

Some practical measures are as follows:

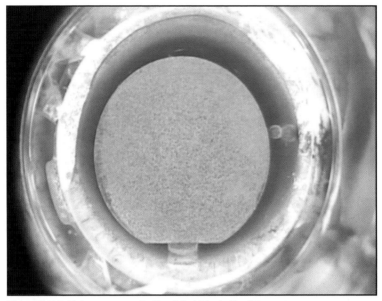

Figure 3-5. Initial surgery resulted in air bubbles in the AC.

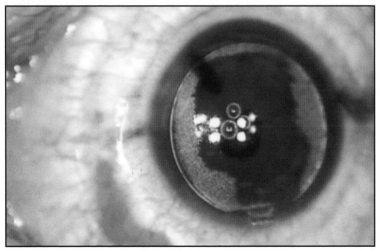

Figure 3-6. VISX laser was used for the excimer procedure. Dimming the microscope light and asking the patient to look down did not lead to successful tracking.

- Decrease flap diameter on the fellow eye by 0.5 mm.
- During excimer laser treatment, dim the microscope light and ask the patient to look down during the tracker registration to drive the bubbles superiorly. This may lead to better exposure of the pupil to the tracker.

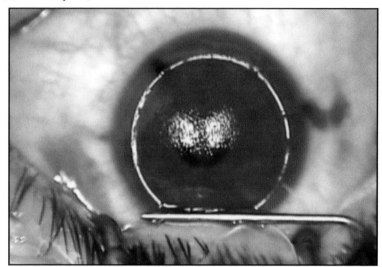

Figure 3-7. Patient was asked to wait before proceeding with excimer laser treatment. The air bubble resorbed partially 1 hour later.

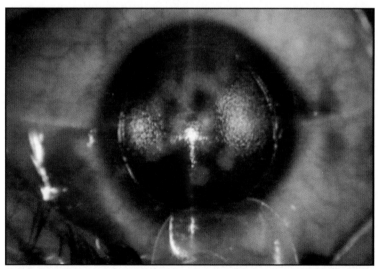

Figure 3-8. Ablation was subsequently performed. On the left eye, the flap diameter was decreased to 8.9 mm. No air bubble was seen in the AC, and the excimer procedure was uneventful. On the first day after surgery, the patient had an uncorrected distance visual acuity of 20/20 in each eye, with LASIK flaps clear and well-centered on slit lamp examination. At his 2-month follow-up visit, uncorrected distance visual acuity was 20/20 in each eye.

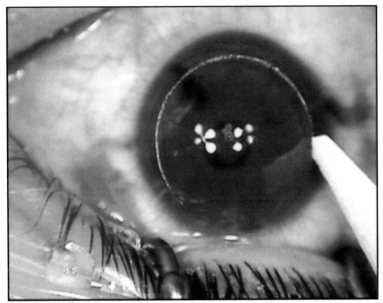

Figure 3-9. Photograph taken at the end of the surgery showing that small air bubbles can be suitable with tracking activation.

- In some cases, the above maneuvers are not successful.
- Waiting for air bubbles to resorb is sometimes the only possible solution. This can take between 30 minutes and several hours.

General Practical Measures in Femtosecond LASIK Surgery

Once air bubbles in AC are detected, the following measures should be taken:

- Continue laser treatment.
- Decrease flap diameter on the fellow eye by 0.3 to 0.5 mm.
- During the excimer procedure, ask the patient during tracker registration to look down and then up.
- Try dimming the microscope light to enlarge the pupil diameter.
- Disable the tracker only in small ametropia (especially with slower lasers).

- Do not turn off the tracker in cases of astigmatism and high ametropia and if using a fast laser avoid a decentered ablation. Waiting for air bubbles to resorb may be the appropriate solution.
- It may take between 30 minutes and several hours for air bubbles to resorb.

PREVENTION OF AIR BUBBLES IN ANTERIOR CHAMBER

Gas bubbles in the AC appear to correlate with femtosecond dissection that is too close to the limbus, which often occurs in smaller corneas, larger flaps, and high applanation pressures. The following are some suggestions to help prevent air bubbles in the AC:

- Select a smaller diameter flap when excessive scleral show is noted after the application of the suction ring.
- Select a smaller flap for the fellow eye and turn the pocket off to prevent the complication from occurring again.

REFERENCES

1. Farjo AA, Sugar A, Schallhorn SC, et al. Femtosecond lasers for LASIK flap creation: a report by the American Academy of Ophthalmology. *Ophthalmology.* 2013;120(3):e5-e20.
2. Soong HK, de Melo Franco R. Anterior chamber gas bubbles during femtosecond laser flap creation in LASIK: video evidence of entry via trabecular meshwork. *J Cataract Refract Surg.* 2012;38(12):2184-2185.
3. Utine CA, Altunsoy M, Basar D. Visante anterior segment OCT in a patient with gas bubbles in the anterior chamber after femtosecond laser corneal flap formation. *Int Ophthalmol.* 2010;30(1):81-84.
4. Srinivasan S, Rootman DS. Anterior chamber gas bubble formation during femtosecond laser flap creation for LASIK. *J Refract Surg.* 2007;23(8):828-830.
5. Moshirfar M, Gardiner JP, Schliesser J, et al. Laser in situ keratomileusis flap complications using mechanical microkeratome versus femtosecond laser: retrospective comparison. *J Cataract Refract Surg.* 2010;36(11):1925-1933.
6. Robert MC, Khreim N, Todani A, Melki SA. Anterior chamber gas bubble emergence pattern during femtosecond LASIK-flap creation. *Br J Ophthalmol.* 2015;99(9):1201-1205.

SUGGESTED READING

Faktorovich E. *Femtodynamics.* Thorofare, NJ: SLACK Inc; 2009.
Shah DN, Melki S. Complications of femtosecond-assisted laser in-situ keratomileusis flaps. *Semin Ophthalmol.* 2014;29(5-6):363-375.

Please see videos on the accompanying website at
www.healio.com/books/lasikvideos

4

Buttonholed Flaps and Vertical Gas Breakthrough

ETIOLOGY AND INCIDENCE OF BUTTONHOLED FLAPS AND VERTICAL GAS BREAKTHROUGH

Femtosecond LASIK

Cavitation bubbles from the femtosecond laser can dissect upwards toward the epithelium and are called *vertical bubble breaks*.[1-3] The bubbles may either stay below Bowman's membrane or break through the epithelium. When the bubbles stay under Bowman's layer, a focal thinning in the flap is noted. If the break is through the epithelium, this is considered a *buttonhole*.

The following 2 types of bubbles have been described:
- Partial bubble breaks characterized by a gray/white appearance.
- Full breaks characterized by a deep black appearance. They are thought to occur due to the dissection of cavitation bubbles into the subepithelial space.

Risk factors include corneal scars, microscopic breaks in Bowman's membrane, and thin flaps, which can lead to accidental vertical gas breakthrough (VGB). Reported VGB incidence varies between 0% with the

Melki SA, Fadlallah A.
LASIK Emergencies: A Video Primer (pp 39-52).
© 2018 SLACK Incorporated.

60 kilohertz (kHz) femtosecond laser (IntraLase [Abbott Medical Optics]) and 1.3% with Femto LDV (Ziemer Ophthalmic Systems).[4,5]

Microkeratome LASIK

A buttonholed flap occurs when the microkeratome blade travels more superficially than intended and enters the epithelium/Bowman's complex. Buttonholes may be partial thickness if they transect Bowman's layer or full thickness if they exit through the epithelium. The incidence of buttonholes ranges between 0.2% and 0.56%.[1,6] No clear etiology has been identified for this complication. Presumed risk factors include the following:

- High keratometric values, although this is not consistent with our experience.
- Previous incisional keratotomy.
- Pre-existing surface lesion (eg, pterygium, corneal scars).

FEMTOSECOND LASIK COMPLICATIONS AND IMMEDIATE SOLUTIONS

Complication #1: Black Vertical Gas Breakthrough in Visual Axis

Video section: 1 minute 58 seconds

Platform: IntraLase FS60 (kHz) (Abbott Medical Optics)

Flap diameter: 9.3 mm

Flap target depth: 100 microns (μm)

The initial surgery on the right eye resulted in black VGB in the visual axis (video 4; time: 1 minute 58 seconds; Figures 4-1, 4-2, and 4-3).

Some practical measures are as follows:

- Continue the femtosecond laser treatment to avoid a partial flap.
- Assess the position of the VGB within the flap.
- The flap with black VGB affecting the visual axis should not be lifted and surgery should be aborted.

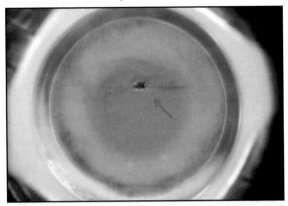

Figure 4-1. Initial surgery resulted in black VGB in the visual axis (red arrow).

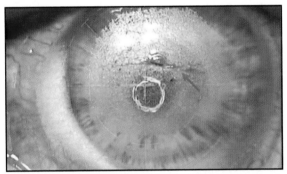

Figure 4-2. Photograph showing black VGB in the visual axis (red arrow).

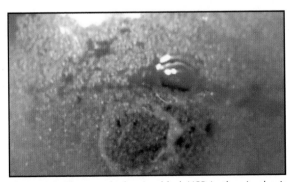

Figure 4-3. Photograph showing black VGB in the visual axis (red arrow). Surgery was aborted. Surgery in the fellow eye was uneventful. One month later, the right eye underwent LASIK surgery. At the 2-month follow-up visit, uncorrected distance visual acuity was 20/20 in each eye.

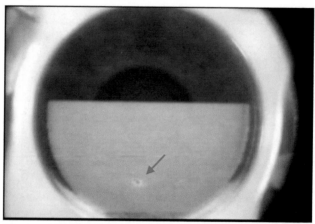

Figure 4-4. Initial surgery resulted in white/gray VGB in the paracentral pupillary area (red arrow).

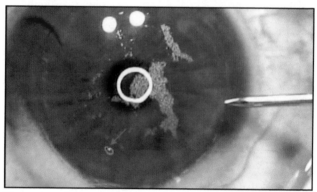

Figure 4-5. Photograph showing white/gray VGB in the paracentral pupillary area (red arrow).

Complication #2: White/Gray Paracentral Vertical Gas Breakthrough

Video section: 2 minutes 10 seconds

Platform: IntraLase FS60 kHz

Flap diameter: 9.3 mm

Flap target depth: 100 μm

The initial surgery on the right eye resulted in white/gray paracentral pupillary VGB (video 4; time: 2 minutes 10 seconds; Figures 4-4, 4-5, and 4-6).

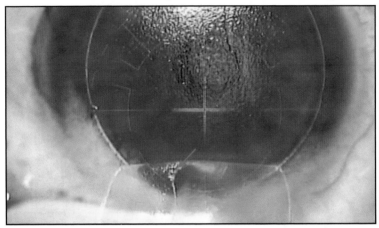

Figure 4-6. Flap lift did not result in a full-thickness buttonhole (red arrow) (see Figure 4-15). Excimer laser treatment was uneventful. Surgery was uneventful in the fellow eye.

Some practical measures are as follows:

- Continue the femtosecond laser treatment.
- Start gentle mechanical flap dissection around the VGB area.
- Assess the position of air bubbles within the flap; white VGB is at lower risk of tearing during a flap lift.
- Consider using flap forceps to lift the flap and prevent any tear.

Complication #3: Black Peripheral Vertical Gas Breakthrough

Video section: 2 minutes 55 seconds
Platform: IntraLase FS60 kHz
Flap diameter: 9.3 mm
Flap target depth: 100 μm

The initial surgery on the right eye resulted in black VGB in the periphery (video 4; time: 2 minutes 55 seconds; Figures 4-7, 4-8, 4-9, and 4-10).

Some practical measures are as follows:

- Continue the femtosecond laser treatment.
- Start gentle mechanical flap dissection around the VGB area.
- Assess the position of air bubbles within the flap.

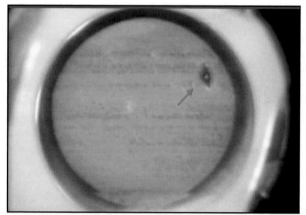

Figure 4-7. Initial surgery resulted in black VGB in the periphery (red arrow).

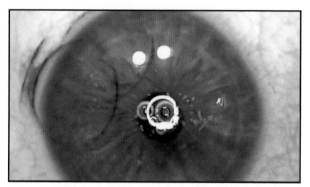

Figure 4-8. Photograph showing black VGB in the periphery (red arrow).

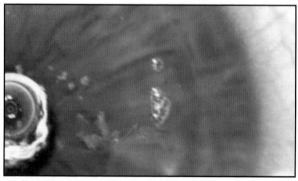

Figure 4-9. Photograph showing black VGB in the periphery (red arrow).

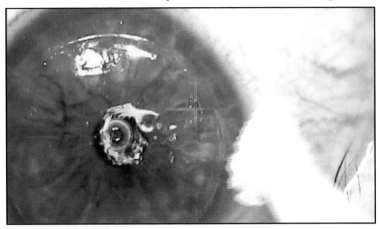

Figure 4-10. Flap lift resulted in small buttonhole in the periphery (red arrow). Excimer laser treatment was uneventful. Surgery was uneventful in the fellow eye.

- A flap with peripheral black VGB not involving the visual axis may be lifted carefully if the surgeon determines that a buttonhole in this area is acceptable.
- Consider using flap forceps to gently lift the flap to prevent any tear.

Complication #4: White Peripheral Vertical Gas Breakthrough

Video section: 4 minutes 32 seconds
Platform: IntraLase FS60 kHz
Flap diameter: 9.3 mm
Flap target depth: 100 μm

The initial surgery resulted in white VGB in the periphery (video 4; time: 4 minutes 32 seconds; Figures 4-11, 4-12, 4-13, and 4-14).

Some practical measures are as follows:
- Continue the femtosecond laser treatment.
- Start gentle mechanical flap dissection around the VGB area.
- Assess the position of air bubbles within the flap; white VGB is at lower risk of tearing during a flap lift.
- Consider using flap forceps to lift the flap and prevent any tear.

The initial surgery on the left eye resulted in white VGB in the periphery (see Figures 4-6 and 4-7). A flap lift and excimer laser treatment in the right eye and left eye (see Figures 4-8 and 4-9) were uneventful. At the patient's

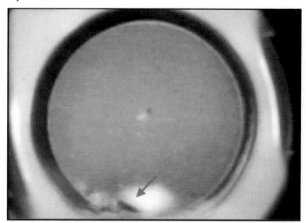

Figure 4-11. Initial surgery resulted in white VGB in the periphery (red arrow).

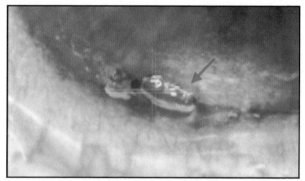

Figure 4-12. Photograph showing white VGB in the periphery (red arrow).

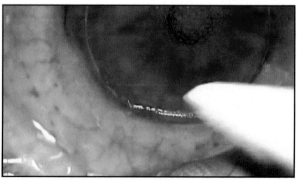

Figure 4-13. Flap lift and excimer laser treatment were uneventful. Surgery was uneventful in the fellow eye.

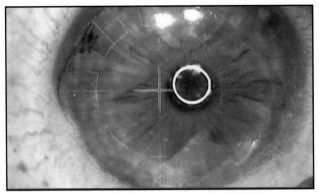

Figure 4-14. Corneal appearance at the end of the procedure.

2-month follow-up visit, the uncorrected distance visual acuity was 20/15 in each eye and topography pattern was within normal limits in the left eye.

General Practical Measures in Femtosecond LASIK Surgery

Once VGB is detected, the following should occur:
- Continue the femtosecond laser treatment to avoid a partial flap.
- Assess the position of air bubbles within the flap.
- Do not lift flaps with VGB (black and/or white) to avoid affecting the visual axis.
- Full central breaks (buttonhole) should not be lifted.
- Full peripheral breaks (buttonhole) may be lifted and excimer laser treatment attempted.
- Partial bubble breaks in the periphery could be carefully lifted.

MICROKERATOME LASIK COMPLICATIONS AND IMMEDIATE SOLUTIONS

Complication #5: Buttonhole

Video section: 6 minutes 10 seconds
Platform: Hansatome (Bausch + Lomb)
Flap diameter: 9.5 mm

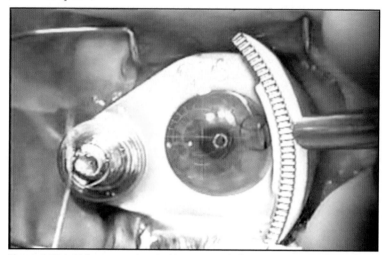

Figure 4-15. Initial surgery using the Hansatome platform.

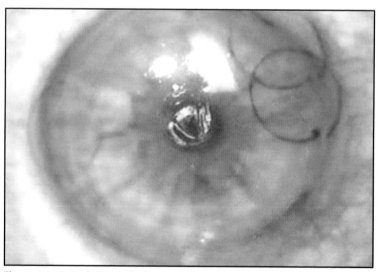

Figure 4-16. Irregular corneal reflex noted after the keratome pass.

Flap target depth: 120 μm

The initial surgery on the right eye resulted in a central buttonhole (video 4; time: 6 minutes 10 seconds; Figures 4-15, 4-16, and 4-17).

Some practical measures are as follows:

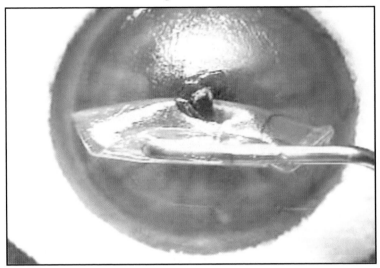

Figure 4-17. Photograph showing the buttonhole during flap lifting. Surgery was aborted, and a surface refractive procedure was planned several weeks later (as discussed in Chapter 15).

- Abort the surgery.
- Plan for a future surface refractive procedure.

Complication #6: Buttonhole Associated With Pterygium

Video section: 8 minutes 5 seconds
Platform: Hansatome
Flap diameter: 9.5 mm
Flap target depth: 120 μm

The initial surgery on the right eye resulted in a central buttonhole (video 2; time: 8 minutes 5 seconds; Figure 4-18).

Some practical measures are as follows:

- Abort the surgery.
- Plan for a future surface refractive procedure.

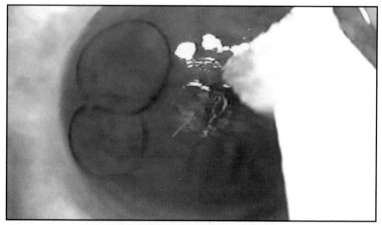

Figure 4-18. Initial surgery resulted in a buttonhole (red arrow). Pterygium is seen in the nasal area.

General Practical Measures in Microkeratome LASIK Surgery

Once a buttonhole is detected, the following should occur:

- Abort the surgery.
- Follow the algorithm to determine the best course of action (Figure 4-19).[6]

PREVENTION OF BUTTONHOLED FLAPS AND VERTICAL GAS BREAKTHROUGH

Femtosecond LASIK

A careful slit lamp examination prior to surgery should reveal areas of scarring that are typically the precursors to vertical bubble breaks. Eyes that have had previous radial keratotomy surgery are also at higher risk of vertical gas dissection. The incidence of splaying the radial keratotomy incision can be high and may be due to gas breakthrough or from the mechanical lifting. Surface ablation may be a safer approach in these situations.

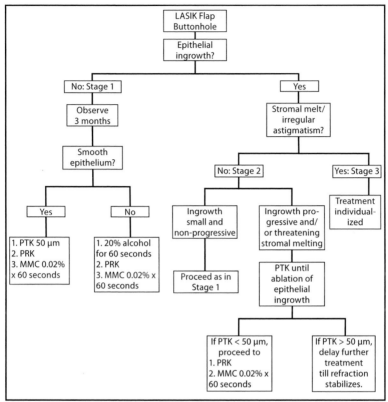

Figure 4-19. Algorithm.

Microkeratome LASIK

Avoid cutting the flap if the intraocular pressure is low due to low suction. Set the microkeratome to a deeper cutting depth if keratometry readings show evidence of a steep cornea, assuming that the amount of intended myopic correction to be treated allows such modification. Most refractive surgeons follow such an approach, setting the cut-off point at 46 to 48 diopters (D), although no definitive supportive study exists in the literature.

REFERENCES

1. Melki S, Azar DT. LASIK complications: etiology, management, and prevention. *Surv Ophthalmol.* 2001;46(2):95-116.
2. Srinivasan S, Herzig S. Sub-epithelial gas breakthrough during femtosecond laser flap creation for LASIK. *Br J Ophthalmol.* 2007;91(10):1373.
3. Shah DN, Melki S. Complications of femtosecond-assisted laser in-situ keratomileusis flaps. *Semin Ophthalmol.* 2014;29(5-6):363-375.
4. Prakash G, Agarwal A, Kumar DA, et al. Femtosecond sub-bowman keratomileusis: a prospective, long-term, intereye comparison of safety and outcomes of 90- versus 100-µm flaps. *Am J Ophthalmol.* 2011;152(4):582-590.
5. Pietilä J, Huhtala A, Jääskeläinen M, Jylli J, Mäkinen P, Uusitalo H. LASIK flap creation with the Ziemer femtosecond laser in 787 consecutive eyes. *J Refract Surg.* 2010;26(1):7-16.
6. Harissi-Dagher M, Todani A, Melki S. Laser in situ keratomileusis buttonhole: classification and management algorithm. *J Cataract Refract Surg.* 2008;34(11):1892-1899.

SUGGESTED READING

Muñoz G, Albarrán-Diego C, Sakla HF, Pérez-Santonja JJ, Alió JL. Femtosecond laser in situ keratomileusis after radial keratotomy. *J Cataract Refract Surg.* 2006;32(8):1270-1275.

Muñoz G, Albarrán-Diego C, Sakla HF, Javaloy J. Femtosecond laser in situ keratomileusis for consecutive hyperopia after radial keratotomy. *J Cataract Refract Surg.* 2007;33(7):1183-1189.

Please see videos on the accompanying website at

www.healio.com/books/lasikvideos

Opaque Bubble Layer

Etiology and Incidence of Opaque Bubble Layer

Opaque bubble layer (OBL) varies in incidence depending on the particular femtosecond laser that is used. Some femtosecond laser systems have programs that create a decompression pocket or channel that facilitates gas escape during the raster pass.[1-3] In some cases, gas can still collect in the stroma and lead to an OBL.[1-3]

Cavitation bubbles formed during flap creation can expand into a cleavage plane at the stromal interlamellar space, which connects to the surface via the side cut. It is hypothesized that when the laser energy is too high (causing excessive bubbles) or too low (resulting in an inadequate pocket to vent the bubbles), microplasma bubbles can travel in errant directions, push apart collagen fibrils around them, and expand into the created space.[4] This is especially true in cases where the pocket/channel is turned off and no meniscus is present.[4] It is also thought that older patients have denser collagen in the peripheral cornea and sclera compared with younger patients, which may not allow bubbles to exit the periphery.[4] Steeper, thicker corneas, small flap, and hard-docking technique have been associated with more OBLs.[4]

Reported OBL incidence varies between 3.69% on WaveLight FS200 (Alcon Labs) and 52.5% on IntraLase FS60 kilohertz (kHz) (Abbott Medical

Melki SA, Fadlallah A.
LASIK Emergencies: A Video Primer (pp 53-61).
© 2018 SLACK Incorporated.

Optics).[5] Studies using the IntraLase 60 kHz femtosecond laser found that 52.5% developed an OBL of various severities.[5] Forty percent were with a hard pattern, and 12.5% were with a soft pattern (under pocket-on mode).[5-8] Studies on eyes undergoing WaveLight FS200 femtosecond LASIK found an average of 3.69% OBL in the flap area in the group with 1.7 mm channel length and 6.06% OBL in the group with 1.3 mm channel length.[6] Studies on the VisuMax 500 kHz femtosecond laser (Carl Zeiss Meditec Inc) shows that the incidence of OBL was 5%. Studies on FEMTO LDV Z6 (Ziemer Ophthalmic Systems) shows that the incidence of OBL was 2%.[9]

FEMTOSECOND LASIK COMPLICATIONS AND IMMEDIATE SOLUTIONS

Complication #1: Opaque Bubble Layer in Visual Axis

Video section: 1 minute 5 seconds

Platform: IntraLase FS60 kHz

Flap diameter: 9.3 mm

Flap target depth: 100 microns (μm)

The initial surgery resulted in OBL reaching the visual axis (video 5; time: 1 minute 5 seconds; Figures 5-1, 5-2, and 5-3).

Some practical measures are as follows:

- Downward pressure with a spatula over the involved area after flap lifting may facilitate tracker registration and pachymetry measurement.

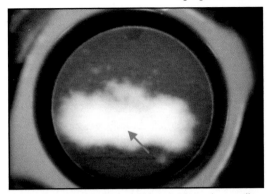

Figure 5-1. Initial surgery resulted in OBL in the pupillary area (red arrow).

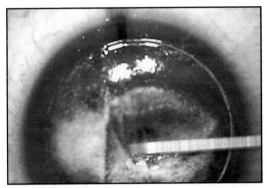

Figure 5-2. Downward pressure with a spatula over the involved stromal area was exerted to express the air out and to facilitate tracker registration and pachymetry measurement.

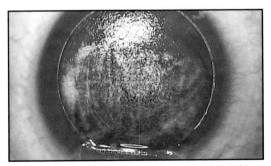

Figure 5-3. Excimer laser treatment (VISX STAR S4 [Abbott Medical Optics]) was then uneventful.

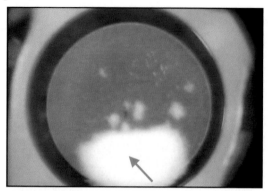

Figure 5-4. Initial surgery resulted in OBL in the superior area reaching the pupillary zone (red arrow).

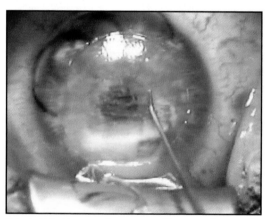

Figure 5-5. Downward pressure with a spatula over the involved area was exerted to spread the bubbles into adjacent corneal layers and to facilitate tracker registration and pachymetry measurement.

Complication #2: Opaque Bubble Layer Superiorly Extending to Visual Axis

Video section: 2 minutes 7 seconds

Platform: WaveLight FS200

Flap diameter: 9.3 mm

Flap target depth: 100 μm

The initial surgery resulted in OBL reaching the visual axis (video 5; time: 2 minutes 7 seconds; Figures 5-4, 5-5, and 5-6).

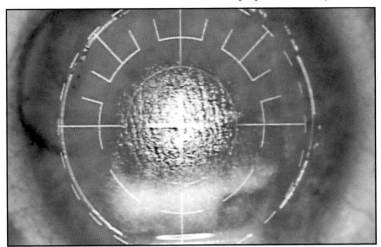

Figure 5-6. Excimer laser treatment (WaveLight EX500 [Alcon Labs]) was then uneventful.

Some practical measures are as follows:
- As stated previously, downward pressure with a spatula over the involved area may facilitate tracker registration and pachymetry measurement.

Complication #3: Opaque Bubble Layer Superiorly With Vertical Gas Breakthrough

Video section: 3 minutes 9 seconds
Platform: WaveLight FS200
Flap diameter: 9.3 mm
Flap target depth: 100 μm

The initial surgery resulted in OBL reaching the visual axis. A vertical gas breakthrough can also be seen in the superior area. Flap adhesion was noted superiorly (video 5; time: 3 minutes 9 seconds; Figures 5-7, 5-8, 5-9, 5-10, 5-11, and 5-12).

Some practical measures are as follows:
- Downward pressure with a spatula over the involved area may facilitate tracker registration.
- Firm dissection and using flap forceps may be helpful to release the adhesion.
- Measuring the optical zone with a caliber may be necessary to ensure an adequate stromal bed exposure for excimer laser treatment.
- Reducing the optical zone to 6 mm may facilitate laser treatment.

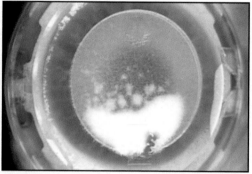

Figure 5-7. Initial surgery resulted in OBL in the superior area reaching the pupillary zone. A vertical gas breakthrough can also be seen in the superior area.

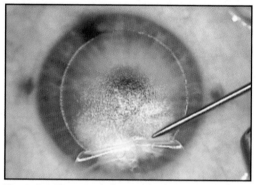

Figure 5-8. Photograph showing flap adhesion superiorly.

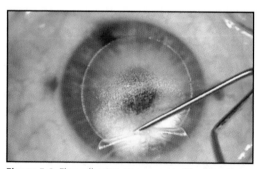

Figure 5-9. Flap adhesion was separated by firm dissection using the flap lifter. Downward pressure over the involved area was exerted to spread the bubbles into adjacent corneal layers and to facilitate tracker registration and pachymetry measurement.

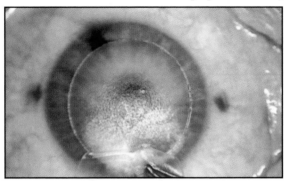

Figure 5-10. Flap adhesion was separated by firm dissection using flap forceps.

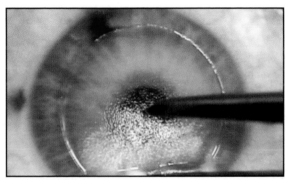

Figure 5-11. Optical zone was then evaluated from the adherent area to the center of the pupil to guarantee at least a 6-mm treatment zone.

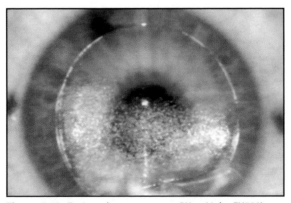

Figure 5-12. Excimer laser treatment (WaveLight EX500) was then uneventful.

General Practical Measures in Femtosecond LASIK Surgery

Once OBL is detected, the following should occur:

- Continue laser treatment.
- OBL may interfere with the tracker or the iris registration of the excimer.
- After lifting the flap, press firmly with a spatula to dissipate some of the trapped gas from the stroma to help pupillary tracking and pachymetry measurement.
- OBL usually dissipates within minutes to hours.
- OBL may lead to a tighter flap adhesion, which can result in flap tears if not dissected carefully.
- Consider using the flap-lifting forceps to release the adherence between the flap and the underlying stoma.
- Always ensure adequate pupil recognition by the tracker to avoid decentered ablations.

PREVENTION OF OPAQUE BUBBLE LAYER

OBL has not been shown to affect refractive outcomes with the excimer laser. OBL may be avoided by performing a *soft dock*, which pertains to docking the patient interface enough on the suction ring to leave a ring of tear meniscus through which the cavitation bubbles can escape. It also prevents mechanical pressure that may seal the vertical pocket where bubbles are usually collected.

REFERENCES

1. Mrochen M, Wullner C, Krause J, Klafke M, Donitzky C, Seiler T. Technical aspects of the WaveLight FS200 femtosecond laser. *J Refract Surg.* 2010;26(10):S833-S840.
2. Kanellopoulos AJ, Asimellis G. Three-dimensional LASIK flap thickness variability: topographic central, paracentral and peripheral assessment, in flaps created by a mechanical microkeratome (M2) and two different femtosecond lasers (FS60 and FS200). *Clin Ophthalmol.* 2013;7:675-683.
3. Faktorovich E. *Femtodynamics.* Thorofare, NJ: SLACK Inc; 2009.
4. Jung HG, Kim J, Lim TH. Possible risk factors and clinical effects of an opaque bubble layer created with femtosecond laser–assisted laser in situ keratomileusis. *J Cataract Refract Surg.* 2015;41(7):1393-1399.
5. Liu CH Sun CC, Hui-Kang Ma D, et al. Opaque bubble layer: incidence, risk factors, and clinical relevance. *J Cataract Refract Surg.* 2014;40(3):435-440.
6. Kanellopoulos JA, Asimellis G. Essential opaque bubble layer elimination with novel LASIK flap settings in the FS200 femtosecond laser. *Clin Ophthalmol.* 2013;7:765-770.
7. Shah SA, Stark WJ. Mechanical penetration of a femtosecond laser-created laser-assisted in situ keratomileusis flap. *Cornea.* 2010;29(3):336-338.
8. Salomão MQ, Wilson SE. Femtosecond laser in laser in situ keratomileusis. *J Cataract Refract Surg.* 2010;36(6):1024-1032.
9. Pietilä J, Huhtala A, Mäkinen P, Salmenhaara K, Uusitalo H. Laser-assisted in situ keratomileusis flap creation with the three-dimensional, transportable Ziemer FEMTO LDV model Z6 I femtosecond laser. *Acta Ophthalmol.* 2014 Nov;92(7):650-655.

SUGGESTED READING

Shah DN, Melki SA. Complications of femtosecond-assisted laser in-situ keratomileusis flaps. *Semin Ophthalmol.* 2014;29(5-6):363-375.

Please see videos on the accompanying website at
www.healio.com/books/lasikvideos

6

Free Flaps

ETIOLOGY AND INCIDENCE OF FREE FLAPS

Femtosecond LASIK

A *free flap* or a *cap* is a rare but significant complication that can occur with femtosecond LASIK. This can happen during flap manipulation rather than during flap creation. Following its creation, the corneal flap can be inadvertently severed from the hinge in the process of lifting, positioning, and refloating. On occasion, a tear may happen at the hinge leading to a free flap. Risk factors include the following:

- Tight adherence of the flap to the closed lid speculum due to flap dehydration resulting from a longer than typical procedure.
- A thin corneal flap.

Some of the potential complications of free flap include irregular astigmatism, recurrent flap dislodgement, and complete flap loss. Studies show a rate of less than 0.5% of true free flap during femtosecond LASIK.[1,2]

Microkeratome LASIK

A free flap results from unintended complete dissection of the corneal flap. Flat corneas (K < 42 diopters [D]) are more prone to this complication. Often, a free flap is thinner than intended. Intraoperative factors leading to a free flap include the following:

Melki SA, Fadlallah A.
LASIK Emergencies: A Video Primer (pp 63-72).
© 2018 SLACK Incorporated.

- Inadequate suction ring placement.
- Lack of synchronization between translational keratome movement and oscillatory blade movement.
- Malposition and misadjustment of the thickness foot-plate or the "stop" mechanism during assembly of microkeratomes (early models of certain horizontal microkeratomes eg, Bausch + Lomb's ACS keratome).
- Microkeratome jam, preventing microkeratome head reversal to free the cap. This might prompt the surgeon to release the suction, thus lifting the instrument with an incarcerated flap, resulting in a free flap.

The reported incidence of true free flap during micokeratome LASIK ranges from 0.01% to 1% in large sample studies.[3]

FEMTOSECOND LASIK COMPLICATIONS AND IMMEDIATE SOLUTIONS

Complication #1: Free Flap

Video section: 0 minutes 26 seconds

Platform: IntraLase FS60 kilohertz (kHz) (Abbott Medical Optics)

Flap diameter: 9.3 mm

Flap target depth: 90 microns (μm)

The initial surgery on the right eye resulted in air bubbles in the anterior chamber. Radial gentian violet marks were applied using an optical zone marker at the intersection of the flap edge and corneal bed. The flap was carefully lifted, and excimer laser ablation was applied. In the process of repositioning the flap back onto the ablated corneal bed, its tight adherence to the lid speculum resulted in a full-thickness detachment of the flap from its superior hinge (video 6; time: 0 minutes 26 seconds; Figures 6-1, 6-2, 6-3, 6-4, 6-5, 6-6, and 6-7).

Some practical measures are as follows:

- Reposition the free flap using the fiduciary marks.
- Place a 10-0 nylon suture at the 9 o'clock position with an air knot to minimize any torque, irregular astigmatism, or decentration tension.
- Place a contact lens.

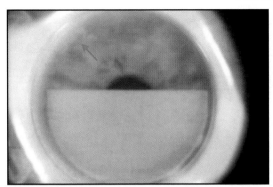

Figure 6-1. Initial surgery resulted in air bubbles in the anterior chamber (red arrow).

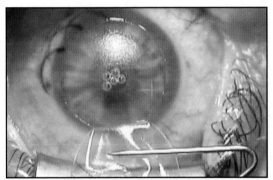

Figure 6-2. Flap positioned on lid speculum. Air bubbles led to a longer procedure and flap dehydration.

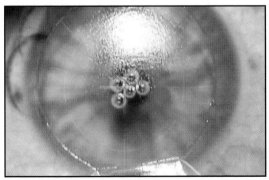

Figure 6-3. Air bubbles made tracking difficult and led to a longer procedure and flap dehydration.

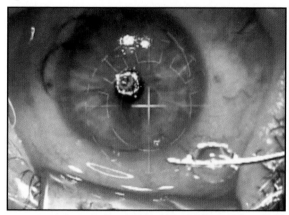

Figure 6-4. While the flap was being pushed down with the irrigation cannula, its tight adherence to the lid speculum resulted in a full detachment of the superiorly located hinge.

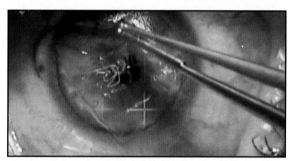

Figure 6-5. Flap was realigned using the previously placed fiduciary marks.

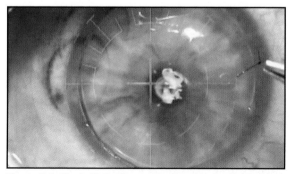

Figure 6-6. Single 10-0 nylon suture was placed at the 9 o'clock position with an air knot to keep the suture loose with minimal vector force on the flap and the corneal bed.

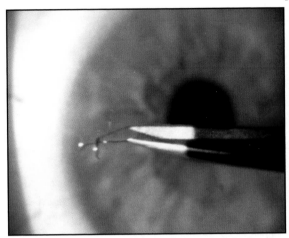

Figure 6-7. On the first postoperative day, the free flap was clear and well-centered. The suture was removed under direct visualization at the slit lamp without complications. At 3 months postoperatively, the free flap was clear and well-centered. The corrected distance visual acuity was 20/20 with a refraction of -2.50 sphere (preoperative monovision target).

General Practical Measures in Femtosecond LASIK Surgery

Once a free flap is detected, the following should occur:

- If the exposed stroma is of the appropriate size and quality, laser ablation treatment can proceed as planned. If the exposed stroma is smaller than treatment optical zone, abort the procedure to allow proper flap alignment. Surface excimer treatment can be planned after 1 week.

- If the free flap is intact, the placement of fiduciary marks at the interface edge between the corneal flap and the peripheral cornea usually allows the surgeon to replace the free flap in its original position.

- The flap is then removed and placed epithelial side down between 2 moist methylcellulose sponges.

- When the markings are not placed or are effaced during irrigation, improper orientation may result in irregular astigmatism.

- The placement of a 10-0 nylon suture is the best method to secure the flap. Proposed alternatives include the placement of a contact lens and pressure patching. These are not as secure as a suture and may lead to flap loss.

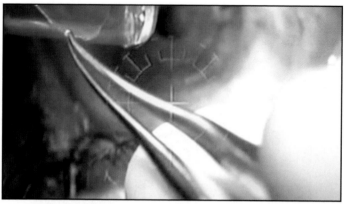

Figure 6-8. Initial surgery resulted in a free flap. The flap was retrieved inside the microkeratome head.

MICROKERATOME LASIK COMPLICATIONS AND IMMEDIATE SOLUTIONS

Complication #2: Free Flap

Video section: 2 minutes 10 seconds

Platform: M2 Microkeratome (Moria)

Flap diameter: 9.5 mm

Flap target depth: 120 μm

The initial surgery on the right eye resulted in a free flap (video 6; time: 2 minutes 10 seconds; Figures 6-8, 6-9, 6-10, and 6-11).

Some practical measures are as follows:

- Try to locate the flap inside the microkeratome and assess whether it is intact.

- When the markings are not placed or are effaced during irrigation, the technique described by Todani et al can be used to adequately reposition the free flap by marking the free flap with gentian violet and then using it to adequately orient the flap (Figure 6-12).

- For the subsequent steps, refer to Complication #1 with femtosecond LASIK.

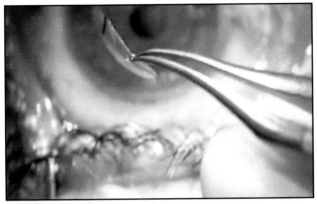

Figure 6-9. Flap was repositioned on the stromal bed.

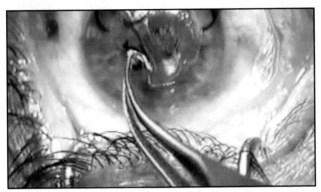

Figure 6-10. Proper flap alignment using fiduciary marks.

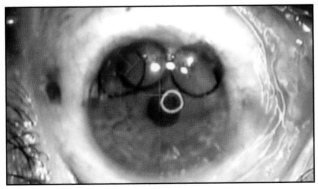

Figure 6-11. Flap alignment at the end of the surgery.

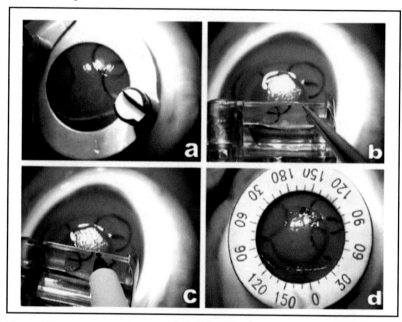

Figure 6-12. Creation of a free LASIK flap with an automated microkeratome. (A) Following placement of a longitudinal corneal incision at the proposed hinge site, the vacuum shaft is aligned so the arrow on the suction ring points superiorly (12 o'clock position). (B) The free flap is inspected on the superior surface of the microkeratome head. (C) A dot of gentian violet is applied to the most peripheral epithelial edge of the flap on the side facing the surgeon. (D) After the flap is retrieved, it is placed on the corneal bed, epithelial side up. A Mendez Degree Gauge is placed on the cornea with the 0 degree reference mark aligned at the 12 o'clock position (corresponding to the position of the arrow on the suction ring).

General Practical Measures in Microkeratome LASIK Surgery

Once a free flap is detected, the following should occur:

- Try to locate the flap inside the microkeratome and assess whether it is intact.

- When the markings are not placed or are effaced during irrigation, the Todani et al technique can be used to adequately reposition free flap by applying a dot of gentian violet on the free flap (peripheral epithelial edge; see Figure 6-12).

- For the remaining steps, refer to Complication #1 with femtosecond LASIK.

- If the free flap cannot be retrieved, the corneal epithelium is allowed to heal. The excimer laser treatment should be aborted and retreatment should be deferred until refractive stability is achieved.

PREVENTION OF FREE FLAP

Femtosecond LASIK

Because a free flap is commonly due to difficulty with lifting the flap, flap lifting technique modification may help to decrease the incidence of free flap. For a difficult flap lift, dissection should be conducted by lifting smaller flap portions one at a time. The tip of the lifting spatula should be parallel to the stroma rather than pointed upwards to avoid a tear. Additionally, being cognizant of the instrument for dissection and its tilt, speed, and rotation can also be important to avoid inadvertent hinge detachment. Minimizing patient factors such as eye movement or squeezing can also be key to preventing this complication.

Microkeratome LASIK

The incidence of free flaps may be reduced if the surgeon ensures adequate suction, inspects the blades, adjusts the plate thickness according to corneal curvature, and pays attention to the following guidelines:

- Avoid cutting the flap if the intraocular pressure is low.
- Use larger suction rings in flat corneas.
- Inspect the microkeratome blade under the operating microscope before engaging it in the suction ring to rule out manufacturing or other preoperative damage.

LASIK Enhancement

Identify the hinge prior to lifting the flap. Surgeons who routinely use superior hinges may not recognize that an old flap has a nasal hinge and may therefore tear it inadvertently. Areas of old epithelial ingrowth may result in scarring and lead to a thin or melted flap that could easily tear upon lifting.

REFERENCES

1. Pietilä J, Huhtala A, Jääskeläinen M, Jylli J, Mäkinen P, Uusitalo H. LASIK flap creation with the Ziemer femtosecond laser in 787 consecutive eyes. *J Refract Surg.* 2010;26(1):7-16.
2. Todani A, Al-Arfaj K, Melki SA. Repositioning free laser in situ keratomileusis flaps. *J Cataract Refract Surg.* 2010;36(2):200-202.
3. Melki SA, Azar DT. LASIK complications: etiology, management, and prevention. *Surv Ophthalmol.* 2001;46(2):95-116.

SUGGESTED READING

Choi CJ, Melki S. Loose anchoring suture to secure a free flap after laser in situ keratomileusis. *J Cataract Refract Surg.* 2012;38(7):1127-1129.

Shah DN, Melki SA. Complications of femtosecond-assisted laser in-situ keratomileusis flaps. *Semin Ophthalmol.* 2014;29(5-6):363-375.

Please see videos on the accompanying website at

www.healio.com/books/lasikvideos

7

Flap Tears

Etiology and Incidence of Flap Tears

Femtosecond LASIK

Flap tears occur with the femtosecond laser mostly during flap dissection rather than during flap creation. Femtosecond-created flaps are more resistant to lifting compared with the microkeratome-created flaps. The risk of tear is even higher with thinner flaps. On occasion, a tear may occur at the hinge, leading to a free flap. Flap tears can also occur during the dissection of flaps with a vertical gas breakthrough (VGB). The incidence of torn flaps is approximately between 0.1% and 0.4% in eyes with femtosecond-assisted flaps; similar percentages are found in eyes treated with microkeratome LASIK.[1,2]

Microkeratome LASIK

Flap tears can also occur with microkeratome LASIK, and are mainly associated with concomitant complications, such as thin and irregular flaps.

Melki SA, Fadlallah A.
LASIK Emergencies: A Video Primer (pp 73-82).
© 2018 SLACK Incorporated.

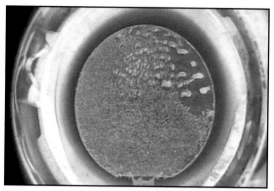

Figure 7-1. Initial surgery resulted in an irregular flap cut pattern.

FEMTOSECOND LASIK COMPLICATIONS AND IMMEDIATE SOLUTIONS

Complication #1: Flap Tear During Flap Dissection

Video section: 0 minutes 15 seconds

Platform: IntraLase FS60 kilohertz (kHz) (Abbott Medical Optics)

Flap diameter: 9.3 mm

Flap target depth: 90 microns (μm)

The initial surgery resulted in a flap tear in the periphery during flap dissection (video 6; time: 0 minutes 15 seconds; Figures 7-1, 7-2, 7-3, and 7-4).

Some practical measures are as follows:

- Assess the position of the flap tear within the flap.
- A small peripheral flap tear may be lifted. Dissect the flap toward the tear followed by the rest of the flap until it is entirely free.
- In cases of severe adherence, surgery should be aborted and a plan for a future surface refractive procedure should be established.
- Place a contact lens.

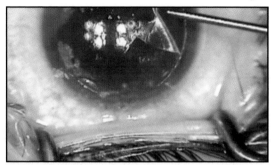

Figure 7-2. Dissection resulted in a flap tear at 9 o'clock on an unusual thin flap.

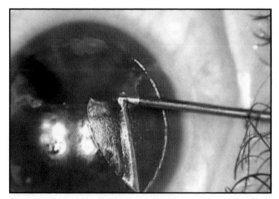

Figure 7-3. Further dissection resulted in extension of the tear. The flap was repositioned, and the surgery was aborted.

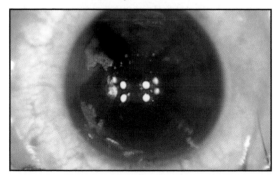

Figure 7-4. Flap was repositioned, and the surgery was aborted. A surface refractive procedure was performed 1 week later. At 3 months postoperatively, the flap was clear and well-centered with no signs of epithelial ingrowth. The uncorrected visual acuity was 20/20.

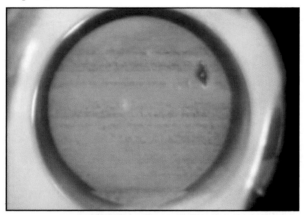

Figure 7-5. Initial surgery resulted in a black VGB in the periphery.

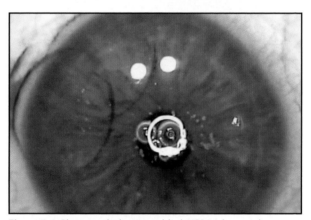

Figure 7-6. Photograph showing a black VGB in the periphery.

Complication #2: Flap Tear on Vertical Gas Breakthrough

Video section: 2 minutes 20 seconds
Platform: IntraLase FS60 kHz
Flap diameter: 9.3 mm
Flap target depth: 90 μm

The initial surgery resulted in a black VGB in the periphery and a flap tear during dissection (video 7; time: 2 minutes 20 seconds; Figures 7-5, 7-6, and 7-7).

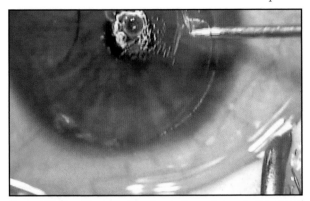

Figure 7-7. Flap lift resulted in a tear in the periphery in the area of VGB. Excimer laser treatment was uneventful.

Some practical measures are as follows:
- Assess the position of the flap tear within the flap.
- A small peripheral flap tear may be lifted. Dissect the flap toward the tear followed by the rest of the flap until it is entirely free.
- Apply excimer laser treatment.
- Place a contact lens.

Complication #3: Iatrogenic Flap Tear During Dissection

Video section: 4 minutes 16 seconds
Platform: IntraLase FS60 kHz
Flap diameter: 9.3 mm
Flap target depth: 90 µm
   The initial surgery resulted in a flap tear during dissection (video 7; time: 4 minutes 16 seconds; and Figures 7-8, 7-9, and 7-10).
   Some practical measures are as follows:
- Assess the position of the flap tear within the flap.
- A small peripheral flap tear may be lifted. Dissect the flap toward the tear followed by the rest of the flap until it is entirely free.
- Apply excimer laser treatment.
- Place a contact lens.

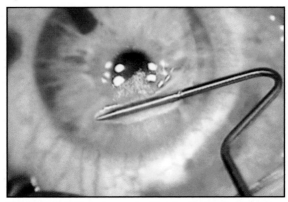

Figure 7-8. Initial surgery resulted in a flap tear during dissection.

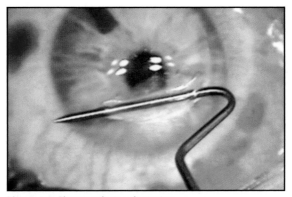

Figure 7-9. Flap tear during dissection.

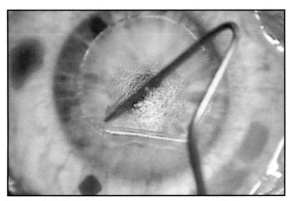

Figure 7-10. Excimer laser treatment was uneventful.

General Practical Measures in Femtosecond LASIK Surgery

Once a free tear is detected, the following should occur:

- Assess the position of the flap tear within the flap.
- Large flap tears affecting the visual axis should be repositioned. If the procedure is aborted, surface ablation is the safest approach to complete the treatment.
- Small peripheral flap tears may be lifted. One can dissect the flap toward the tear followed by the rest of the flap until it is entirely free.
- In cases of a free flap, put a loose anchoring suture to secure the flap after completion of the stromal ablation.

MICROKERATOME LASIK COMPLICATIONS AND IMMEDIATE SOLUTIONS

Complication #4: Irregular Thin Torn Flap

Video section: 8 minutes 57 seconds
Platform: Hansatome (Bausch + Lomb)
Flap diameter: 9.5 mm
Flap target depth: 120 µm

The initial surgery resulted in an irregular torn flap construction due to poor suction occurring at two-thirds the distance across the planned cut (Figures 7-11 and 7-12).

Some practical measures are as follows:

- Assess the available space for the excimer laser treatment.
- Plan for a future surface refractive procedure if the extent of the stromal bed created is not adequate to apply the excimer treatment.

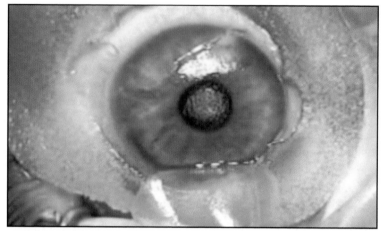

Figure 7-11. Irregular flap construction due to poor suction. Stromal bed is inadequate for the excimer laser treatment.

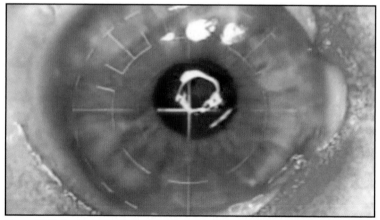

Figure 7-12. Surgery was aborted, and future refractive surgery was planned.

General Practical Measures in Microkeratome LASIK Surgery

Once a flap tear is detected, the following should occur:
- Assess the available space for the excimer laser treatment.
- Plan for a future surface refractive procedure if the extent of the stromal bed created is not adequate to apply the excimer laser treatment.

PREVENTION OF FLAP TEARS

Femtosecond LASIK

Because a flap tear is commonly due to difficulty with lifting the flap, optimizing energy settings and technique may help to decrease its incidence. As discussed in Chapter 6, for a difficult flap lift, dissection should be limited to smaller flap portions at a time. The tip of the lifting spatula should be parallel to the stroma rather than pointed upwards. Peripheral tags can be prevented by increasing the side cut energy, by decreasing the raster energy, or by refining flap lift techniques. Additionally, being cognizant of the instrument for dissection and its tilt, speed, and rotation can also be important to avoid tag creation. Ensuring adequate suction and minimizing patient factors such as eye movement or squeezing can be key to preventing this complication.

Microkeratome LASIK

As with free flaps, the incidence of flap tears may be reduced if the surgeon ensures adequate suction, inspects the blades, adjusts the plate thickness according to corneal curvature, and pays attention to the following guidelines:

- Avoid cutting the flap if the intraocular pressure is low.
- Inspect the microkeratome blade under the operating microscope before engaging it in the suction ring to rule out manufacturing or other preoperative damage.

REFERENCES

1. Ang M, Mehta JS, Rosman M, et al. Visual outcomes comparison of 2 femto-second laser platforms for laser in situ keratomileusis. *J Cataract Refract Surg.* 2013;39(11):1647-1652.
2. Moshirfar M, Gardiner JP, Schliesser J, et al. Laser in situ keratomileusis flap com-plications using mechanical microkeratome versus femtosecond laser: retrospective comparison. *J Cataract Refract Surg.* 2010;36(11):1925-1933.

SUGGESTED READING

Shah DN, Melki SA. Complications of femtosecond-assisted laser in-situ keratomileusis flaps. *Semin Ophthalmol.* 2014;29(5-6):363-375.

Please see videos on the accompanying website at

www.healio.com/books/lasikvideos

8

Incomplete Flaps

ETIOLOGY AND INCIDENCE OF INCOMPLETE FLAPS

Femtosecond LASIK

An incomplete flap may happen with femtosecond LASIK if suction proves to be unsuccessful, despite repeated attempts after an initial aborted pass. It may also occur if the tear meniscus, debris, ink marks, or epithelial defect shields an area of the flap from the laser ablation. The incidence of incomplete flaps with femtosecond LASIK is approximately 0.03%.[1,2]

Microkeratome LASIK

Incomplete flaps may occur with microkeratome LASIK after loss of suction. Microkeratome jamming due to either electrical failure or mechanical obstacles may also result in incomplete flaps. Lashes, drape, loose epithelium, and precipitated salt from the irrigating solution have been recognized as possible impediments to smooth keratome head progression. Incomplete flaps also occur when the gear advancement mechanism jams or is inadequate. The incidence of incomplete flaps with microkeratome LASIK varies between 0.23% and 1.2%.[3]

Melki SA, Fadlallah A.
LASIK Emergencies: A Video Primer (pp 83-104).
© 2018 SLACK Incorporated.

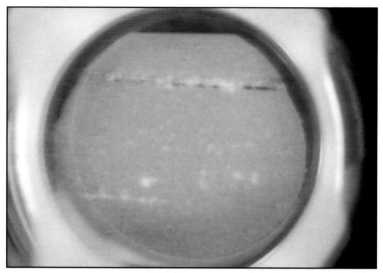

Figure 8-1. Initial surgery resulted in a suction loss during the raster cut. The raster and side cuts were not repeated in this case.

FEMTOSECOND LASIK COMPLICATIONS AND IMMEDIATE SOLUTIONS

Complication #1: Incomplete Flap (Unable to Lift)

Video section: 0 minutes 6 seconds

Platform: IntraLase FS60 kilohertz (kHz) (Abbott Medical Optics)

Flap diameter: 9.3 mm

Flap target depth: 100 microns (μm)

The initial surgery resulted in a partial suction loss. Laser treatment was continued. Adherence was found during dissection at the place where suction was lost (video 8; time: 0 minutes 6 seconds; Figures 8-1 and 8-2).

Some practical measures are as follows:

- Discontinue the laser treatment immediately and repeat the raster cut.
- Start the mechanical flap dissection in front of and behind the suspected uncut zone (place where suction was lost during the first raster cut).
- Blunt dissection and the use of flap forceps may release adherence.
- Extensive adherence may result in a flap tear with blunt dissection.

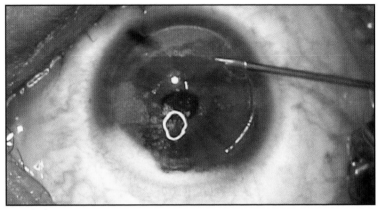

Figure 8-2. Flap lifting revealed adherence at the same place where suction was lost. Surgery was aborted, and the patient underwent a surface refractive procedure 9 days later.

- Abort the procedure.
- Plan for a future surface refractive procedure.

Complication #2: Incomplete Flap (Unable to Lift)

Video section: 1 minute 53 seconds
Platform: WaveLight FS200 (Alcon Labs)
Flap diameter: 9.3 mm
Flap target depth: 100 μm

The initial surgery resulted in an irregular flap cut pattern. Laser treatment was continued. The flap was unable to be lifted (video 2; time: 1 minute 53 seconds; Figures 8-3 and 8-4).

Some practical measures are as follows:

- An irregular raster cut pattern may be due to a deeper stromal cut.
- Abort the procedure.
- Plan for a future surface refractive procedure.

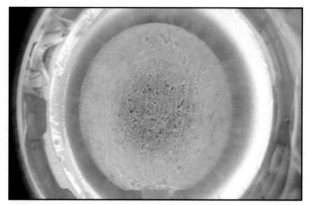

Figure 8-3. Initial surgery resulted in an irregular raster and site cut configuration.

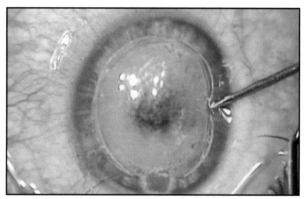

Figure 8-4. Flap lifting was not possible. Surgery was aborted, and the patient underwent a surface refractive procedure 14 days later.

Complication #3: Incomplete Flap (Debris at Interface; Unable to Lift)

Video section: 5 minutes 18 seconds
Platform: IntraLase FS60 kHz
Flap diameter: 9.3 mm
Flap target depth: 100 µm

The initial surgery resulted in an incomplete flap due to debris at the patient interface. Adherence was found during dissection at the place where the debris was found (video 8; time: 5 minutes 18 seconds; Figures 8-5, 8-6, and 8-7).

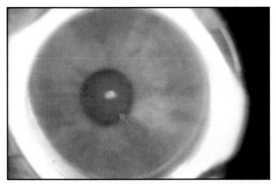

Figure 8-5. Initial surgery showed debris at patient interface (red arrow).

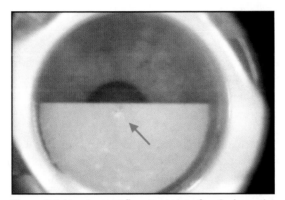

Figure 8-6. Uncut area at flap-stroma interface (red arrow).

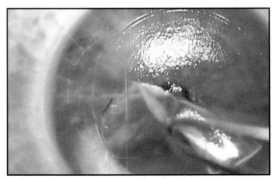

Figure 8-7. Flap lifting was not possible (red arrow). Surgery was aborted, and the patient underwent a surface refractive procedure 7 days later.

Some practical measures are as follows:
- Start the mechanical flap dissection in front of and behind the suspected uncut zone.
- Blunt dissection and the use of flap forceps may release adherence.
- Extensive adherence may result in a flap tear with blunt dissection.
- Abort the procedure.
- Plan for a future surface refractive procedure.

Complication #4: Incomplete Flap (Iatrogenic Epithelial Defect; Unable to Lift)

Video section: 7 minutes 10 seconds

Platform: WaveLight FS200

Flap diameter: 9.3 mm

Flap target depth: 100 μm

The initial surgery resulted in an incomplete flap due to an iatrogenic epithelial defect. Adherence was found during dissection at the place of the epithelial defect (video 8; time: 7 minutes 10 seconds; and Figures 8-8, 8-9, and 8-10).

Some practical measures are as follows:
- Start the mechanical flap dissection in front of and behind the suspected uncut zone.
- Blunt dissection and the use of flap forceps may release adherence.
- Extensive adherence may result in a flap tear with blunt dissection.
- Abort the procedure.
- Plan for a future surface refractive procedure.

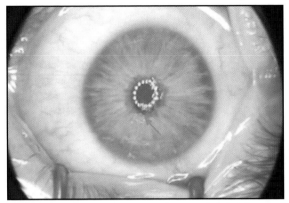

Figure 8-8. Initial surgery showed an epithelial defect (red arrow).

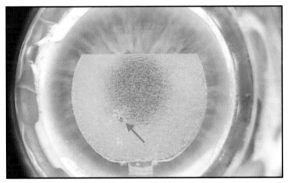

Figure 8-9. Uncut area at the epithelial defect zone (red arrow).

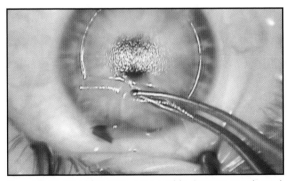

Figure 8-10. Flap lifting was not possible. Surgery was aborted, and the patient underwent a surface refractive procedure 11 days later.

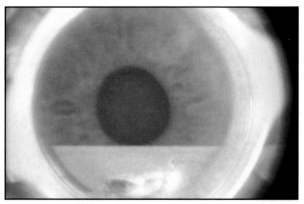

Figure 8-11. Uncut area at the epithelial defect zone.

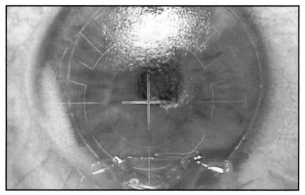

Figure 8-12. Flap lifting showed adherence at the epithelial defect zone.

Complication #5: Incomplete Flap (Iatrogenic Epithelial Defect; Able to Lift)

Video section: 8 minutes 45 seconds

Platform: IntraLase FS60 kHz

Flap diameter: 9.3 mm

Flap target depth: 100 μm

The initial surgery resulted in an incomplete flap due to an iatrogenic epithelial defect. Adherence was found during dissection at the place of the epithelial defect (video 8; time: 8 minutes 45 seconds; Figures 8-11, 8-12, and 8-13).

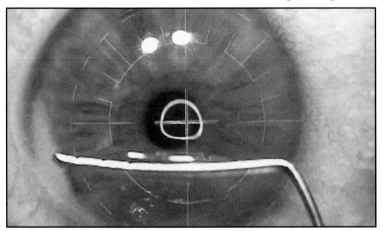

Figure 8-13. Optical zone was reduced to 6 mm, and the excimer laser treatment was applied.

Some practical measures are as follows:
- Start the mechanical flap dissection in front of and behind the suspected uncut zone.
- Blunt dissection and the use of flap forceps may release adherence.
- Assess the available stromal bed for the excimer laser treatment.
- Reduce the optical zone to 6 mm.
- Apply the excimer laser treatment.

Complication #6: Incomplete Flap (Able to Lift With Forceps)

Video section: 10 minutes 10 seconds
Platform: IntraLase FS60 kHz
Flap diameter: 9.3 mm
Flap target depth: 100 μm
The initial surgery resulted in a partial suction loss. Laser treatment was not discontinued. A second raster cut was successfully attempted. Adherence was found during dissection at the place where suction was lost (video 8; time: 10 minutes 10 seconds; Figures 8-14, 8-15, 8-16, and 8-17).

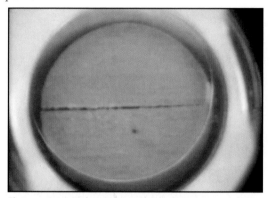

Figure 8-14. Initial surgery resulted in a suction loss during the raster cut.

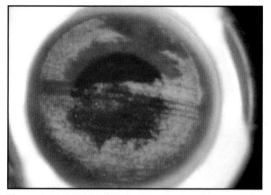

Figure 8-15. Raster and side cuts were repeated.

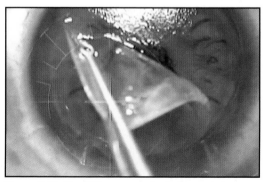

Figure 8-16. Flap lifting revealed adherence at the same place where suction was lost first. Use of forceps to release adherence is recommended.

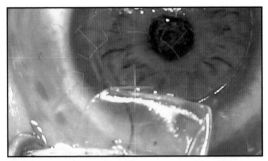

Figure 8-17. Adherence was released, and the excimer laser treatment was applied successfully.

Some practical measures are as follows:
- Discontinue the laser treatment immediately and repeat the raster cut.
- Start the mechanical flap dissection in front of and behind the suspected uncut zone (place where suction was lost during the first raster cut).
- Blunt dissection may result in a flap tear in the area of the incomplete flap.
- Use flap forceps to release adherence.
- Apply the excimer laser treatment.

Complication #7: Incomplete Flap (Able to Lift With Dissection)

Video section: 11 minutes 31 seconds
Platform: IntraLase FS60 kHz
Flap diameter: 9.3 mm
Flap target depth: 100 μm

The initial surgery resulted in a partial suction loss. Laser treatment was discontinued. A second raster cut was successfully attempted. Adherence was found during dissection at the place where suction was lost (video 8; time: 11 minutes 31 seconds; Figures 8-18, 8-19, 8-20, and 8-21).

Some practical measures are as follows:
- Discontinue the laser treatment immediately and repeat the raster cut.
- Start the mechanical flap dissection in front of and behind the suspected uncut zone (place where suction was lost during the first raster cut).
- Blunt dissection may release adherence.
- Apply the excimer laser treatment.

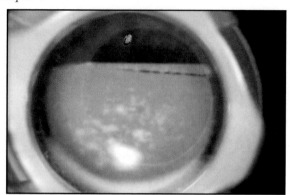

Figure 8-18. Initial surgery resulted in a suction loss during the raster cut.

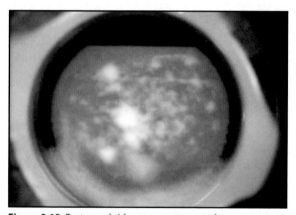

Figure 8-19. Raster and side cuts were repeated.

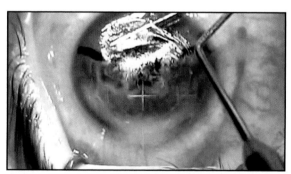

Figure 8-20. Flap lifting revealed adherence at the same place where suction was initially lost.

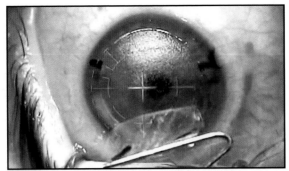

Figure 8-21. Adherence was released by simple dissection, and the excimer laser treatment was applied successfully.

Complication #8: Incomplete Flap (Able to Lift With Use of Vannas Scissors at Edge)

Video section: 12 minutes 37 seconds

Platform: IntraLase FS60 kHz

Flap diameter: 9.3 mm

Flap target depth: 100 µm

The initial surgery on the left eye resulted in an incomplete inferior side construction due to a tear meniscus shields at 6 o'clock after partial suction loss (video 8; time: 12 minutes 37 seconds; Figures 8-22, 8-23, 8-24, and 8-25).

Some practical measures are as follows:

- Start the mechanical flap dissection gently in the cut area toward the uncut zone.
- Try to assess the extent of the uncut area.
- Blunt dissection may result in a flap tear in the area of the incomplete flap.
- Use Vannas scissors to cut the adherent side cut zone.

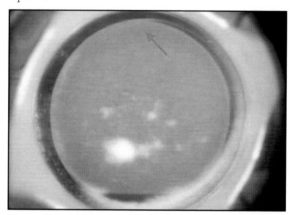

Figure 8-22. Initial surgery resulted in an incomplete inferior side construction due to a torn meniscus shield at 6 o'clock after partial suction loss (red arrow).

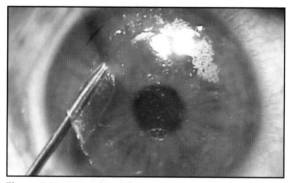

Figure 8-23. Incomplete inferior side construction resistant to dissection.

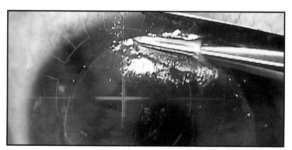

Figure 8-24. Vannas scissors were used to release the adherent side cut.

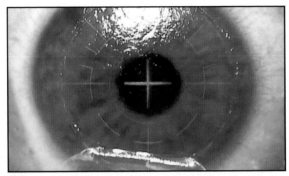

Figure 8-25. Ablation was subsequently performed, and the flap was repositioned.

Complication #9: Incomplete Flap (Ink Mark)

Video section: 15 minutes 27 seconds

Platform: IntraLase FS60 kHz

Flap diameter: 9.3 mm

Flap target depth: 100 µm

The initial surgery resulted in an incomplete flap due to an ink mark used to pinpoint the pupillary center. Adherence was found during dissection at the place of the ink (video 8; time: 15 minutes 27 seconds; Figures 8-26, 8-27, 8-28, and 8-29).

Some practical measures are as follows:

- Start the mechanical flap dissection in front of and behind the suspected uncut zone.
- Blunt dissection and the use of flap forceps may release adherence.
- Extensive adherence may result in a flap tear with blunt dissection.
- Assess the available stromal bed for laser treatment, and apply the excimer laser treatment.

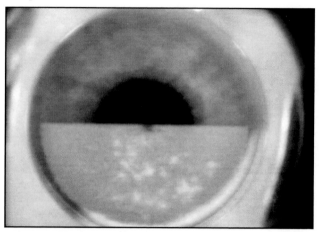

Figure 8-26. Uncut area at the ink zone.

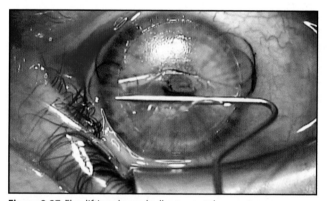

Figure 8-27. Flap lifting showed adherence at the uncut zone.

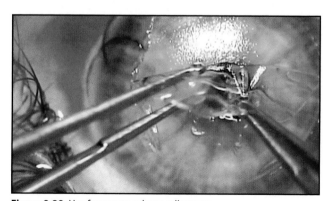

Figure 8-28. Use forceps to release adherence.

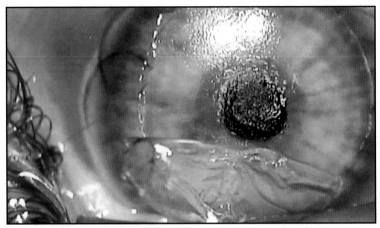

Figure 8-29. Successful flap release and excimer laser treatment.

General Practical Measures in Femtosecond LASIK Surgery

Once incomplete flap is detected, the following should occur:

- Start the mechanical flap dissection in front of and behind the suspected uncut zone.
- Blunt dissection may result in a flap tear in the area of the incomplete flap.
- Use flap forceps to release adherence.
- Use Vannas scissors to cut the adherent side cut zone.
- Abort procedure when extensive adherence and/or irregular raster cut bed are found.
- Plan for a future surface refractive procedure if the excimer laser treatment was not applied.

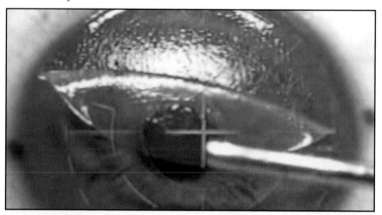

Figure 8-30. Initial surgery resulted in an incomplete flap construction due to suction loss occurring at one-third the distance across the planned cut. Surgery was aborted, and surface refractive procedure was planned 1 week later.

MICROKERATOME LASIK COMPLICATIONS AND IMMEDIATE SOLUTIONS

Complication #10: Loss of Suction During Microkeratome Pass

Video section: 17 minutes 32 seconds
Platform: Hansatome (Bausch + Lomb)
Flap diameter: 9.5 mm
Flap target depth: 120 μm

The initial surgery resulted in an incomplete flap construction due to suction loss occurring at one-third the distance across the planned cut (video 8; time: 17 minutes 32 seconds; Figure 8-30).

Some practical measures are as follows:

- Pause the surgery.
- Assess the available space for the excimer laser treatment.
- Plan for a future surface refractive procedure if the extent of the stromal bed created is not adequate to apply the excimer laser treatment.

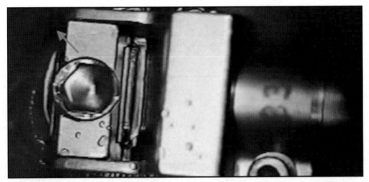

Figure 8-31. Microkeratome jamming due to a mechanical obstacle, resulting in incomplete flap (microkeratome hitting the speculum; red arrow).

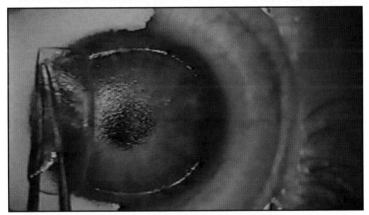

Figure 8-32. Incomplete flap construction due to microkeratome jamming at two-thirds the distance across the planned cut.

Complication #11: Incomplete Flap Due to Mechanical Obstruction

Video section: 17 minutes 52 seconds
Platform: Automated Corneal Shaper (Bausch + Lomb)
Flap diameter: 9.5 mm
Flap target depth: 120 μm

The initial surgery resulted in an incomplete flap construction due to keratome being blocked by the lid speculum occurring at two-thirds the distance across the planned cut (video 8; time: 17 minutes 52 seconds; Figures 8-31, 8-32, and 8-33).

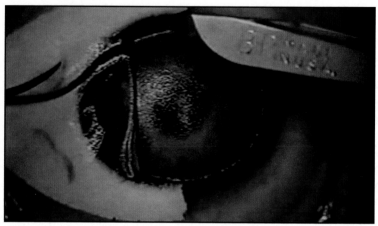

Figure 8-33. Risky maneuver showing blade #15 used to extend the dissection plan. Ablation was subsequently performed.

Some practical measures are as follows:
- Pause the surgery.
- Assess the available space for the excimer laser treatment.
- Avoid manually extending the dissection with a blade, as this can result in a buttonhole during dissection.
- If the laser ablation is performed, the flap should be protected from laser exposure.

General Practical Measures in Microkeratome LASIK Surgery

Once an incomplete flap is detected, the following should occur:
- Pause the surgery.
- Assess the available space for the excimer laser treatment.
- Avoid manually extending the dissection with a blade.
- If the laser ablation is performed, the flap should be protected from laser exposure.
- Abort the procedure in cases involving an irregular bed and/or flap.

Prevention of Incomplete Flaps

Femtosecond LASIK

The main preventable cause of an incomplete flap is suction loss. Careful observation during docking of the patient interface and reposition if necessary can be helpful. Additionally, recognizing preoperative risk factors, such as a deep set orbit, and planning accordingly can also be useful in preventing suction loss. Patients who forcefully squeeze their lids may benefit from additional sedation or the placement of a wire lid speculum. The following interventions may be also helpful in preventing an incomplete flap in femtosecond LASIK:

- Eliminate all patient interface debris using pressurized air dust remover.
- Postpone a flap cut in case of an epithelial defect in the pupillary area.
- Avoid using ink to mark the center of the flap cut.

Microkeratome LASIK

The incidence of incomplete flaps may be reduced if the surgeon ensures adequate suction, inspects the blades, adjusts the plate thickness according to corneal curvature, and pays attention to the following guidelines:

- Avoid cutting the flap if the intraocular pressure is low.
- Use larger suction rings in flat corneas.
- Inspect the microkeratome blade under the operating microscope before engaging it in the suction ring to rule out manufacturing or other preoperative damage.

REFERENCES

1. Davison JA, Johnson SC. Intraoperative complications of LASIK flaps using the IntraLase femtosecond laser in 3009 cases. *J Refract Surg.* 2010;26(11):851-857.
2. Shah DN, Melki SA. Complications of femtosecond-assisted laser in-situ keratomileusis flaps. *Semin Ophthalmol.* 2014;29(5-6):363-375.
3. Nakano K, Nakano E, Oliveira M, Portellinha W, Alvarenga L. Intraoperative microkeratome complications in 47,094 laser in situ keratomileusis surgeries. *J Refract Surg.* 2004;20(5 Suppl):S723-S726.

SUGGESTED READING

Ang M, Mehta JS, Rosman M, et al. Visual outcomes comparison of 2 femtosecond laser platforms for laser in situ keratomileusis. *J Cataract Refract Surg.* 2013;39(11):1647-1652.
Faktorovich E. *Femtodynamics.* Thorofare, NJ: SLACK Inc; 2009.
Melki SA, Azar DT. Lasik complications: etiology, management, and prevention. *Surv Ophthalmol.* 2001;46(2):95-116.
Muñoz G, Albarrán-Diego C, Ferrer-Blasco T, Javaloy J, García-Lázaro S. Single versus double femtosecond laser pass for incomplete laser in situ keratomileusis flap in contralateral eyes: visual and optical outcomes. *J Cataract Refract Surg.* 2012;38(1):8-15.
Rosman M, Hall RC, Chan C, et al. Comparison of efficacy and safety of laser in situ keratomileusis using 2 femtosecond laser platforms in contralateral eyes. *J Cataract Refract Surg.* 2013;39(7):1066-1073.
Syed ZA, Melki SA. Successful femtosecond LASIK flap creation despite multiple suction losses. *Digit J Ophthalmol.* 2014;20(1):7-9.

Please see videos on the accompanying website at
www.healio.com/books/lasikvideos

9

Irregular Flaps

ETIOLOGY AND INCIDENCE OF IRREGULAR FLAPS

Femtosecond LASIK

An irregular flap may happen after suction loss and a repeated flap cut attempt. Another risk factor for an irregular second pass is the disappearance of the transient opaque bubble layer before performing the second femtosecond pass. Irregular flap incidence with femtosecond LASIK is unknown.

Microkeratome LASIK

Irregular flaps (bileveled, bisected, or with a notch) may result from poor suction, damaged microkeratome blades, or irregular oscillation. Irregular flap incidence with microkeratome LASIK varies between 0.09% and 0.2%.[1,2]

Melki SA, Fadlallah A.
LASIK Emergencies: A Video Primer (pp 105-115).
© 2018 SLACK Incorporated.

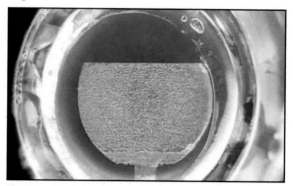

Figure 9-1. Initial surgery resulted in an incomplete flap construction due to suction loss occurring at two-thirds the distance across the planned cut.

FEMTOSECOND LASIK COMPLICATIONS AND IMMEDIATE SOLUTIONS

Complication #1: Double Flap Due to Recut at Different Plane

Video section: 0 minutes 7 seconds
Platform: WaveLight FS200 (Alcon Labs)
Flap diameter: 9.1 mm
Flap target depth: 110 microns (μm)

The initial surgery on the right eye resulted in an incomplete flap construction due to suction loss occurring at one-third the distance across the planned cut. The second pass resulted in complete flap creation. Flap lifting revealed the presence of 2 different flaps that disrupted during dissection (video 9; time: 0 minutes 7 seconds; Figures 9-1, 9-2, 9-3, 9-4, 9-5, 9-6, and 9-7).

Some practical measures are as follows:

- Abort the surgery.
- Try to reconstruct the irregular flap before repositioning.
- Plan for a future surface refractive procedure.

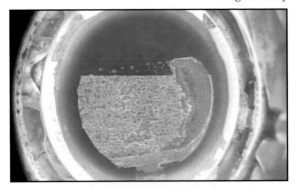

Figure 9-2. Second pass resulted in complete flap creation.

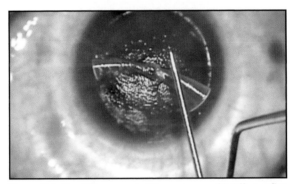

Figure 9-3. Flap lifting revealed the presence of 2 different flap planes.

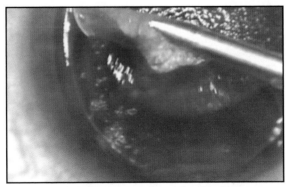

Figure 9-4. Several attempts were undertaken to reconstruct the irregular flap.

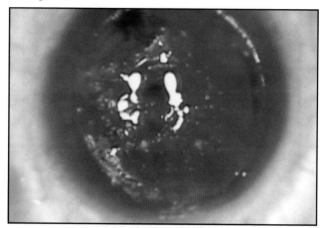

Figure 9-5. Flap was repositioned, and surgery was aborted. On the first day after surgery, the patient had a corrected distance visual acuity of 20/40 with a clear LASIK flap on slit lamp examination. At his 4-month follow-up visit, his corrected distance visual acuity was 20/25 with −2.50 −0.50 × 90 (see Figure 9-14). He underwent a surface refractive procedure with 40 seconds of mitomycin-C 0.02% 1 week later.

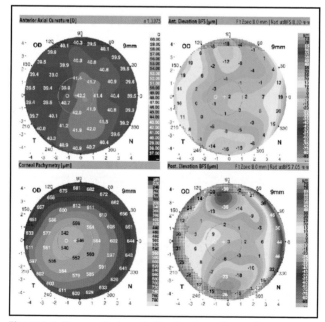

Figure 9-6. Topography 1 week after the aborted procedure.

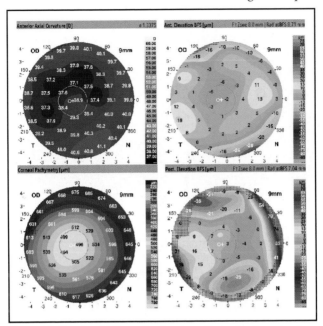

Figure 9-7. Topography 3 months after the surface refractive procedure.

Complication #2: Irregular Flap Secondary to Uneven Cut

Video section: 2 minutes 2 seconds
Platform: IntraLase FS60 kilohertz (kHz) (Abbott Medical Optics)
Flap diameter: 9.3 mm
Flap target depth: 90 µm

The initial surgery resulted in an irregular partial epithelial flap (video 9; time: 2 minutes 2 seconds; Figures 9-8 and 9-9).

Some practical measures are as follows:

- Abort the procedure.
- Try to reconstruct the irregular flap before repositioning.
- Place a contact lens.
- Plan for a future surface refractive procedure.

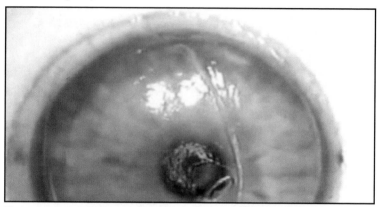

Figure 9-8. Initial surgery resulted in an irregular partial epithelial flap.

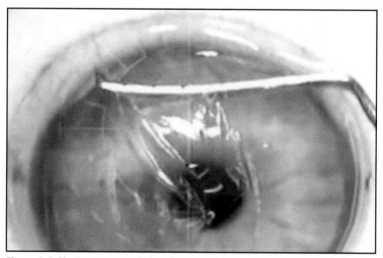

Figure 9-9. Flap was repositioned, and the surgery was aborted. On the first day after surgery, the patient had an uncorrected distance visual acuity of 20/50 with LASIK flaps clear and well-centered on slit lamp examination. At his 1-month follow-up visit, uncorrected distance visual acuity was 20/20. He underwent a surface refractive procedure with 40 seconds mitomycin-C 0.02%. His uncorrected visual acuity 1 month later was 20/20.

Complication #3: Irregular Flap Secondary to Flap Dryness

Video section: 2 minutes 44 seconds

Platform: IntraLase FS60 kHz

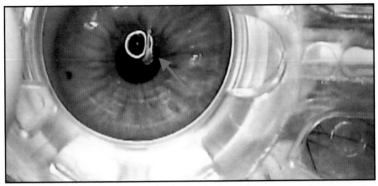

Figure 9-10. Initial surgery showed a dry flap (red arrow).

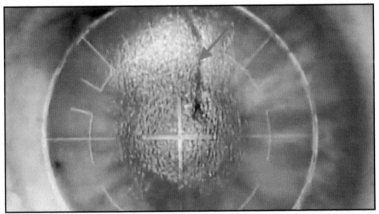

Figure 9-11. Flap lift showed an irregular stromal bed in the paracentral pupillary area (red arrow). The excimer laser treatment was uneventful. At his 2-month follow-up visit, uncorrected distance visual acuity was 20/20.

Flap diameter: 9.3 mm

Flap target depth: 90 μm

The initial surgery resulted in an irregular partial epithelial flap (video 9; time: 2 minutes 44 seconds; Figures 9-10 and 9-11).

Some practical measures are as follows:

- Assess the position of the irregular stromal bed to papillary area.
- Apply the excimer laser treatment if the irregular bed is away from the visual axis.
- Plan for a future surface refractive procedure elsewhere.

General Practical Measures in Femtosecond LASIK Surgery

Once an irregular flap is detected, the following should occur:
- Abort the surgery.
- Try to reconstruct the irregular flap before repositioning.
- Plan for a future surface refractive procedure over the incomplete flap as early as 1 week after the aborted procedure with the application of mitomycin-C to avoid scarring.

MICROKERATOME LASIK COMPLICATIONS AND IMMEDIATE SOLUTIONS

Complication #4: Poor Microkeratome Suction and Irregular Incomplete Flap

Video section: 3 minutes 10 seconds
Platform: Hansatome (Bausch + Lomb)
Flap diameter: 9.5 mm
Flap target depth: 120 μm

The initial surgery resulted in an irregular flap construction due to poor suction occurring at two-thirds the distance across the planned cut (Figures 9-12, 9-13, and 9-14).

Some practical measures are as follows:
- Abort the surgery.
- Try to reconstruct the irregular flap before repositioning.
- Plan for a future surface refractive procedure.

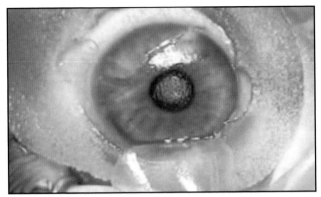

Figure 9-12. Irregular flap construction due to poor suction.

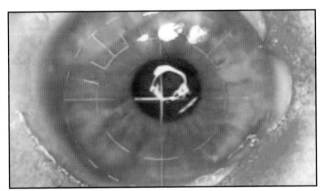

Figure 9-13. Stromal bed was inadequate for the excimer laser treatment.

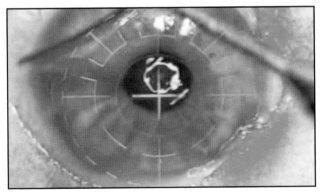

Figure 9-14. Surgery was aborted, and a future refractive surgery was planned.

General Practical Measures in Microkeratome LASIK Surgery

Once irregular flap is detected, the following should occur:
- Abort the surgery.
- Try to reconstruct the irregular flap before repositioning.
- Plan for a future surface refractive procedure over the incomplete flap as early as 1 week after the aborted procedure with the application of mitomycin-C to avoid scarring.

PREVENTION OF IRREGULAR FLAPS

Femtosecond LASIK

Careful observation during docking of the patient interface and repositioning, if necessary, can be helpful to avoid suction loss and the risk of an irregular flap after recuts.

Microkeratome LASIK

The incidence of free flaps may be reduced if the surgeon ensures adequate suction, inspects the blades, adjusts the plate thickness according to corneal curvature, and pays attention to the following guidelines:
- Avoid cutting the flap if the intraocular pressure is low.
- Use larger suction rings in flat corneas.
- Inspect the microkeratome blade under the operating microscope before engaging it in the suction ring to rule out manufacturing or other preoperative damage.

REFERENCES

1. Stulting RD, Carr JD, Thompson KP, et al. Complications of laser in situ keratomileusis for the correction of myopia. *Ophthalmology.* 1999;106(1):13-20.
2. Lin RT, Maloney RK. Flap complications associated with lamellar refractive surgery. *Am J Ophthalmol.* 1999;127(2):129-136.

SUGGESTED READING

Melki SA, Azar DT. LASIK complications: etiology, management, and prevention. *Surv Ophthalmol.* 2001;46(2):95-116.
Shah DN, Melki S. Complications of femtosecond-assisted laser in-situ keratomileusis flaps. *Semin Ophthalmol.* 2014;29(5-6):363-375.

Please see videos on the accompanying website at

www.healio.com/books/lasikvideos

10

Epithelial Defect

ETIOLOGY AND INCIDENCE OF EPITHELIAL DEFECT

Femtosecond and Microkeratome LASIK

An *epithelial defect* is defined as an area of epithelium with a break or loose cells greater than 2 mm. Trauma to the epithelium seems significantly less likely with the femtosecond laser compared with the microkeratome laser. It can still occur during several docking attempts, or especially when inexperienced surgeons have difficulty inserting the dissecting spatula under the flap edge. Epithelial defects tend to occur in patients with predisposing risk factors such as epithelial basement membrane dystrophy or a history of recurrent corneal erosion syndrome. They are also more commonly seen in older patients, in patients with large flap diameters, and with excessive topical anesthetic use. Epithelial defects also tend to occur when lifting the flap for LASIK refractive enhancement. The main advantage of the femtosecond laser is the absence of the keratome rotational movement that can lead to tearing or shearing of the epithelium. The incidence of epithelial defect with femtosecond LASIK is approximately 0.6%,[1-3] while the incidence with microkeratome is between 1% and 8.65%, depending on the type of microkeratome used.[1-3]

Melki SA, Fadlallah A.
LASIK Emergencies: A Video Primer (pp 117-126).
© 2018 SLACK Incorporated.

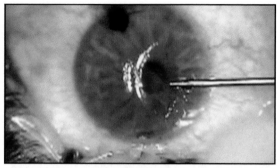

Figure 10-1. Iatrogenic epithelial defect induced during a flap lift.

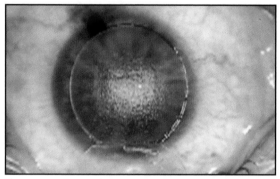

Figure 10-2. Excimer laser treatment was uneventful.

FEMTOSECOND LASIK COMPLICATIONS AND IMMEDIATE SOLUTIONS

Complication #1: Epithelial Defect During Flap Lift

Video section: 0 minutes 5 seconds

Platform: WaveLight FS200 (Alcon Labs)

Flap diameter: 9.3 mm

Flap target depth: 100 microns (μm)

The initial surgery on the left eye resulted in an epithelial defect from an inadvertent epithelial flap lift (video 10; time: 0 minutes 5 seconds; Figures 10-1, 10-2, and 10-3).

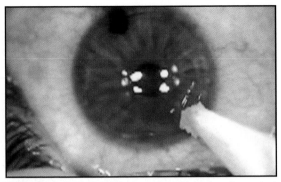

Figure 10-3. Epithelial defect was repositioned, and a contact lens was placed at the end.

Some practical measures are as follows:
- Apply excimer laser treatment.
- Try to reposition the epithelial defect.
- Place a contact lens at the end of the procedure.

Complication #2: Epithelial Defect During Flap Repositioning

Video section: 3 minutes 9 seconds
Platform: WaveLight FS200
Flap diameter: 9.3 mm
Flap target depth: 100 μm

The initial surgery on the left eye resulted in an epithelial defect from flap repositioning (video 10; time: 3 minutes 9 seconds; Figures 10-4 and 10-5).

Some practical measures are as follows:
- Try to reposition the epithelial defect.
- Place a contact lens at the end of the procedure.

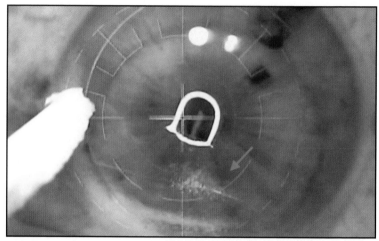

Figure 10-4. Iatrogenic epithelial defect induced during flap repositioning (red arrow).

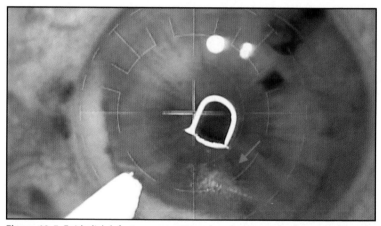

Figure 10-5. Epithelial defect was repositioned, and a contact lens was placed at the end (red arrow).

Complication #3: Epithelial Defect During Flap Lifting for LASIK Enhancement Surgery

Video section: 0 minutes 30 seconds
Platform: WaveLight FS200
Flap diameter: 9.3 mm
Flap target depth: 100 μm

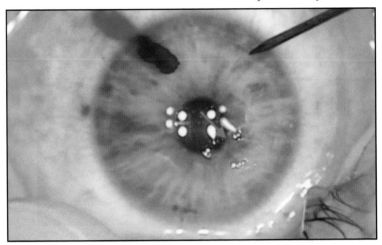

Figure 10-6. Iatrogenic epithelial defect induced during flap lifting (red arrow).

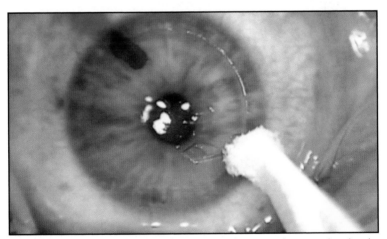

Figure 10-7. Epithelial defect was repositioned, and a contact lens was placed at the end.

The initial surgery on the left eye resulted in an epithelial defect from flap repositioning (video 10; time: 0 minutes 30 seconds; Figures 10-6 and 10-7).

Some practical measures are as follows:

- Try to reposition the epithelial defect.
- Place a contact lens at the end of the procedure.

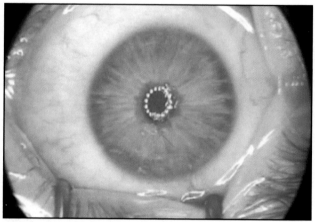

Figure 10-8. Initial surgery showed an epithelial defect (red arrow).

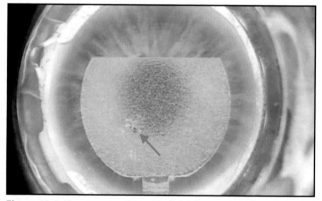

Figure 10-9. Uncut area at the epithelial defect zone (red arrow).

Complication #4: Iatrogenic Epithelial Defect During Docking (Flap Unable to Lift)

Video section: 8 minutes 39 seconds

Platform: WaveLight FS200

Flap diameter: 9.3 mm

Flap target depth: 100 μm

The initial surgery resulted in an incomplete flap due to an iatrogenic epithelial defect. Adherence was found during dissection at the place of the epithelial defect (video 10; time: 8 minutes 39 seconds; Figures 10-8, 10-9, and 10-10).

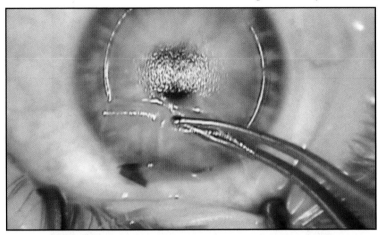

Figure 10-10. Flap lifting was not possible. Surgery was aborted, and the patient underwent a surface refractive procedure 11 days later.

Some practical measures are as follows:

- Start the mechanical flap dissection in front of and behind the suspected uncut zone.
- Blunt dissection and the use of flap forceps may release adherence.
- Extensive adherence may result in a flap tear with blunt dissection.
- Abort the procedure.
- Plan for a future surface refractive procedure.

General Practical Measures in Femtosecond LASIK Surgery

Once an epithelial defect is detected, the following should occur:

- If the epithelial defect happens after femtosecond treatment, one should do as follows:
  - Continue the laser treatment.
  - Lift the flap gently in case an incomplete flap is suspected.
  - Try to reposition the epithelial defect at the end of the procedure.
  - Treat with topical antibiotics and a bandage contact.
- If the epithelial defect happens before femtosecond treatment, refer to Chapter 8.

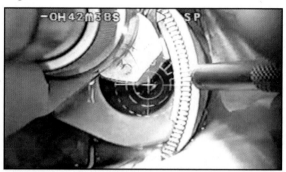

Figure 10-11. Initial surgery was uneventful but resulted in an epithelial defect in the visual axis.

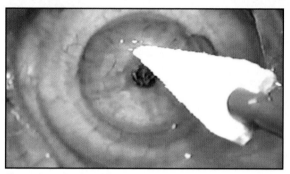

Figure 10-12. Flap lift and excimer laser treatment were uneventful. Epithelial defect was repositioned, and a contact lens was placed.

MICROKERATOME LASIK COMPLICATIONS AND IMMEDIATE SOLUTIONS

Complication #5: Epithelial Defect During Flap Cut

Video section: 10 minutes 14 seconds

Platform: Hansatome (Bausch + Lomb)

Flap diameter: 9.5 mm

Flap target depth: 120 μm

The initial surgery on the right eye resulted in a complete flap cut with an epithelial defect (video 10; time: 10 minutes 14 seconds; Figures 10-11 and 10-12).

Some practical measures are as follows:
- Apply excimer laser treatment.
- Try to reposition the epithelial defect.
- Place a contact lens at the end of the procedure.

General Practical Measures in Microkeratome LASIK Surgery

Once an epithelial defect is detected, the following should occur:
- If the epithelial defect happens without any buttonhole or irregular flap, one should do as follows:
  - Apply excimer laser treatment.
  - Try to reposition the epithelial defect at the end of the procedure.
  - Treat with topical antibiotics and a bandage contact.
- If the epithelial defect happens with a buttonhole, refer to Chapter 4.

PREVENTION OF EPITHELIAL DEFECT

Because the majority of epithelial defects occur in patients with predisposing risk factors, it is important to identify them preoperatively. Patients with asymptomatic epithelial basement membrane dystrophy may still undergo femtosecond LASIK at a much lower risk than with keratome LASIK; however, they should be counseled accordingly. A consideration for surface ablation should be given for patients with a history of symptomatic recurrent corneal erosion syndrome.

REFERENCES

1. Kezirian GM, Stonecipher KG. Comparison of the IntraLase femtosecond laser and mechanical keratomes for laser in situ keratomileusis. *J Cataract Refract Surg.* 2004;30(4):804-811.
2. Feder R, Rapuano C. *The LASIK Handbook: A Case-Based Approach.* Second edition. Philadelphia, PA: Lippincott Williams & Wilkins; 2013.
3. Moshirfar M, Gardiner JP, Schliesser JA, et al. Laser in situ keratomileusis flap complications using mechanical microkeratome versus femtosecond laser: retrospective comparison. *J Cataract Refract Surg.* 2010;36(11):1925-1933.

SUGGESTED READING

Shah DN, Melki S. Complications of femtosecond-assisted laser in-situ keratomileusis flaps. *Semin Ophthalmol.* 2014;29(5-6):363-375.

Please see videos on the accompanying website at

www.healio.com/books/lasikvideos

11

Thin and Thick Flaps

ETIOLOGY AND INCIDENCE OF THIN AND THICK FLAPS

A flap is considered *thin* when the keratome or laser cuts are within or above the 12-microns (μm)-thick Bowman's layer. This is recognized by a shiny reflex on the stromal surface. The use of corneal pachymeter before and after lifting the flap may be helpful in recognizing this occurrence. A measurement below 60 μm is suspicious, as the thickness of the corneal epithelium is approximately 50 μm. The definition of *thick flap* is not clear in the literature, but usually involves flaps with a thickness resulting in a lesser-than-intended residual stromal bed (ie, residual stromal bed < 300 μm after excimer laser treatment). The incidence of thin flaps after LASIK has been reported to vary between 0.3% and 0.75%.[1-3] With femtosecond LASIK, the rate is approximately 0.08%.[1,2] Thick flap incidence is not reported in the literature.

Femtosecond LASIK

Cavitation bubbles from the femtosecond laser can dissect upwards toward the epithelium and may stay below the Bowman's membrane to create a focal or diffuse thinning in the flap. Also, air bubbles may diffuse accidently deeper, creating a thick flap.

Melki SA, Fadlallah A.
LASIK Emergencies: A Video Primer (pp 127-140).
© 2018 SLACK Incorporated.

Microkeratome LASIK

Higher keratometric values offer increased resistance to cutting when applanated, leading to upward or downward movement of the blade, and may result in thin and thick flaps. Also, a lack of synchronization between translational flat keratome movement and oscillatory blade movement results in forward displacement of corneal tissue, leading to thin or thick flaps. Flat corneas may also result in a thin flap, as they could be below the adequate cutting plane in certain locations. Blade positioning in the microkeratome and the preset space for the blade in the microkeratome may affect flap thickness in the absence of an irregular flap shape.

FEMTOSECOND LASIK COMPLICATIONS AND IMMEDIATE SOLUTIONS

Complication #1: Thin Regular Flap

Video section: 0 minutes 5 seconds
Platform: IntraLase FS60 kilohertz (kHz) (Abbott Medical Optics)
Flap diameter: 9.3 mm
Flap target depth: 110 µm

The initial surgery resulted in a thin regular flap that disrupted during flap dissection (video 11; time: 0 minutes 5 seconds; Figures 11-1, 11-2, and 11-3).

Some practical measures are as follows:
- Assess the flap regularity.
- Apply excimer laser treatment with regular flap and an adequate-sized stromal bed.
- Try to reposition the flap and epithelial defect in the best anatomical configuration.
- Place a contact lens.

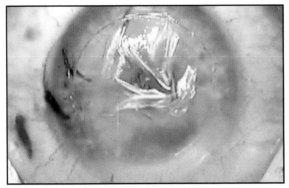

Figure 11-1. Initial surgery resulted in a thin flap with a tear during dissection.

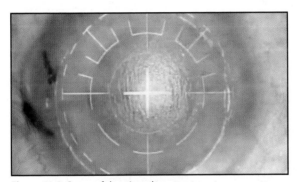

Figure 11-2. Successful excimer laser treatment.

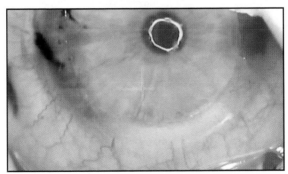

Figure 11-3. Flap was repositioned. At 3 months postoperatively, the flap was clear and well-centered with no signs of epithelial ingrowth.

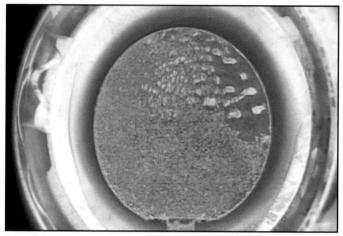

Figure 11-4. Initial surgery resulted in an irregular flap cut pattern.

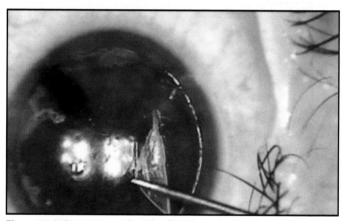

Figure 11-5. Dissection resulted in a flap tear at 9 o'clock on an unusual thin flap.

Complication #2: Localized Thin Regular Flap

Video section: 1 minute 53 seconds

Platform: WaveLight FS200 (Alcon Labs)

Flap diameter: 9.3 mm

Flap target depth: 100 μm

The initial surgery resulted in a thin flap in the periphery with a tear during dissection (video 11; time: 1 minute 53 seconds; Figures 11-4, 11-5, 11-6, and 11-7).

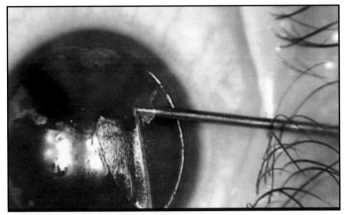

Figure 11-6. Further dissection resulted in an extension of the tear. Flap was repositioned, and the surgery was aborted.

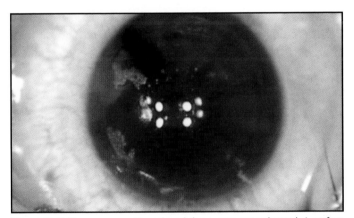

Figure 11-7. Flap was repositioned, and the surgery was aborted. A surface refractive procedure was performed 1 week later.

Some practical measures are as follows:

- Assess the position of the flap tear within the flap.
- A small peripheral flap tear may be lifted. Dissect the flap toward the tear followed by the rest of the flap until it is entirely free.
- In case of severe adherence, surgery should be aborted and one should plan for a future surface refractive procedure.
- Place a contact lens.

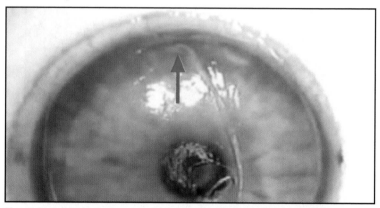

Figure 11-8. Initial surgery resulted in a thin flap. The red arrow shows the intersection between a full-thickness and an epithelial flap. Flap was repositioned, and the surgery was aborted. A surface refractive procedure was performed 1 week later.

Complication #3: Thin Irregular Flap

Video section: 3 minutes 52 seconds
Platform: IntraLase FS60 kHz (Abbott Medical Optics)
Flap diameter: 9.3 mm
Flap target depth: 110 µm
   The initial surgery resulted in a thin irregular flap (partial epithelial flap; video 11; time: 3 minutes 52 seconds; Figure 11-8).
   Some practical measures are as follows:
- Assess the flap regularity.
- Abort the procedure when dealing with an irregular flap.
- Place a contact lens.
- Plan for a future refractive procedure.

Complication #4: Thick Regular Flap

Video section: 6 minutes 19 seconds
Platform: WaveLight FS200
Flap diameter: 9.3 mm
Flap target depth: 100 µm
   The initial surgery resulted in a thick regular flap (video 11; time: 6 minutes 19 seconds; Figures 11-9, 11-10, 11-11, and 11-12).

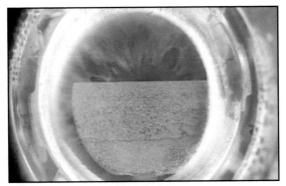

Figure 11-9. Initial surgery resulted in an irregular flap cut pattern.

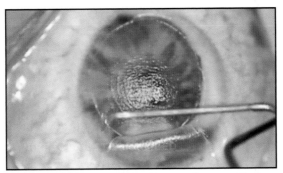

Figure 11-10. Flap lifting showed an irregular stromal bed cut pattern resulting in a thick regular flap.

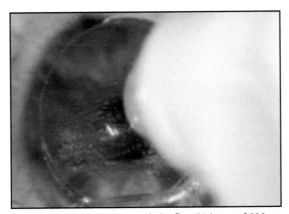

Figure 11-11. Ultrasound revealed a flap thickness of 200 µm and a residual stromal bed of 260 µm in case treatment is undertaken.

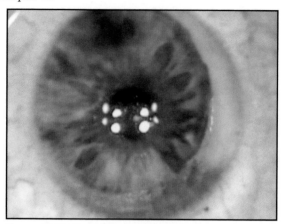

Figure 11-12. Flap was repositioned, and the surgery was aborted. A surface refractive procedure was performed 1 week later.

Some practical measures are as follows:
- Assess the flap and stromal bed regularity.
- Perform corneal pachymetry.
- Abort the procedure if the residual stromal bed will be < 300 μm after the excimer laser treatment.
- Plan for a future refractive procedure.

Complication #5: Thick Irregular Flap

Video section: 7 minutes 12 seconds
Platform: WaveLight FS200
Flap diameter: 9.3 mm
Flap target depth: 100 μm

The initial surgery resulted in a thick irregular flap pattern that was unable to be lifted (video 11; time: 7 minutes 12 seconds; Figures 11-13 and 11-14).

Some practical measures are as follows:
- Abort the procedure.
- Plan for a future refractive procedure.

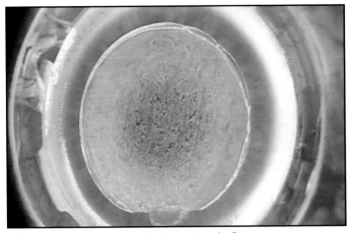

Figure 11-13. Initial surgery resulted in an irregular flap cut pattern.

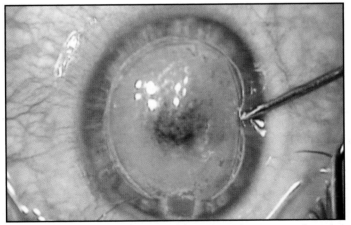

Figure 11-14. Flap was unable to be lifted, and the surgery was aborted. A surface refractive procedure was performed 2 weeks later.

General Practical Measures in Femtosecond LASIK Surgery

Once thin or thick flaps are detected, the following should occur:
- Assess the flap and stromal bed regularity.
- Perform corneal pachymetry.
- Assess the available space for excimer laser treatment.

- Apply excimer laser treatment with thin regular flaps performed under Bowman's layer and with an adequate-sized stromal bed.
- Try to reposition the flap and epithelial defect in the best anatomical configuration.
- Place a contact lens.
- Abort the procedure if the extent of the stromal bed created is not adequate to apply the excimer laser treatment.
- Abort the procedure if the residual stromal bed will be <300 μm after the excimer laser treatment.
- Plan for a future refractive procedure.

Microkeratome LASIK Complications and Immediate Solutions

Complication #5: Thin Regular Flap

Video section: 8 minutes 1 second
Platform: Amadeus II (Ziemer Ophthalmic Systems)
Flap diameter: 9.5 mm
Flap target depth: 120 μm

The initial surgery resulted in a thin regular flap (video 11; time: 8 minutes 1 second; Figures 11-15, 11-16, and 11-17).

Some practical measures are as follows:

- Assess the flap regularity.
- Apply excimer laser treatment with regular flap and an adequate-sized stromal bed.
- Try to reposition the flap in the best anatomical configuration.
- Place a contact lens.

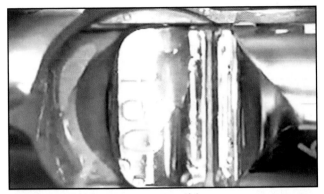

Figure 11-15. Initial surgery was uneventful.

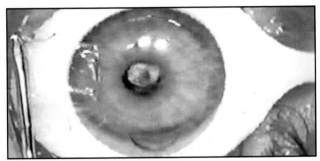

Figure 11-16. Surgery resulted in a thin regular flap. Excimer laser treatment was applied.

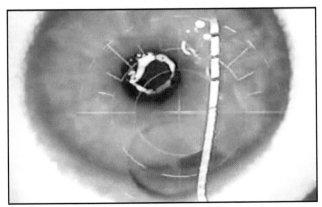

Figure 11-17. Flap was repositioned.

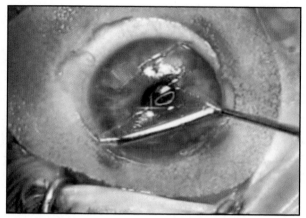

Figure 11-18. Thin irregular flap construction due to poor suction. The stromal bed is inadequate for excimer laser treatment.

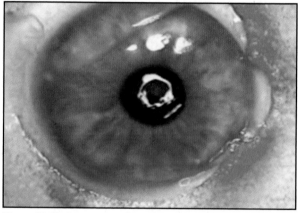

Figure 11-19. Surgery was aborted, and a future refractive surgery was planned.

Complication #6: Thin Irregular Flap

Video section: 8 minutes 47 seconds
Platform: Hansatome (Bausch + Lomb)
Flap diameter: 9.5 mm
Flap target depth: 120 μm

The initial surgery resulted in an irregular torn flap construction due to poor suction occurring at two-thirds the distance across the planned cut (Figures 11-18 and 11-19).

Some practical measures are as follows:
- Assess the available space for excimer laser treatment.
- Abort the procedure and plan for a future surface refractive procedure if the extent of the stromal bed created is not adequate to apply the excimer laser treatment.

General Practical Measures in Microkeratome LASIK Surgery

Once thin or thick flaps are detected, the following should occur:
- Assess the flap and stromal bed regularity.
- Perform corneal pachymetry.
- Assess the available space for excimer laser treatment.
- Apply excimer laser treatment with thin regular flaps and an adequate-sized stromal bed.
- Try to reposition the flap and epithelial defect in the best anatomical configuration.
- Place a contact lens.
- Abort the procedure if the extent of the stromal bed created is not adequate to apply the excimer laser treatment.
- Abort the procedure if the residual stromal bed will be < 300 μm after the excimer treatment.
- Plan for a future refractive procedure.

PREVENTION OF THIN AND THICK FLAPS

Femtosecond LASIK

Thin flaps are usually due to technical issues within the femtosecond laser, and are beyond a surgeon's control. However, ensuring adequate suction and minimizing patient factors such as eye movement or squeezing can help to prevent this complication.

Microkeratome LASIK

The incidence of thin flaps may be reduced if the surgeon ensures adequate suction, inspects the blades, adjusts the plate thickness according to corneal curvature, and pays attention to the following guidelines:

- Avoid cutting the flap if the intraocular pressure is low.
- Inspect the microkeratome blade under the operating microscope before engaging it in the suction ring to rule out manufacturing or other preoperative damage.

REFERENCES

1. Melki SA, Azar DT. LASIK complications: etiology, management, and prevention. *Surv Ophthalmol.* 2001;46(2):95-116.
2. Ang M, Mehta JS, Rosman M, et al. Visual outcomes comparison of 2 femtosecond laser platforms for laser in situ keratomileusis. *J Cataract Refract Surg.* 2013;39(11):1647-1652.
3. Moshirfar M, Gardiner JP, Schliesser J, et al. Laser in situ keratomileusis flap complications using mechanical microkeratome versus femtosecond laser: retrospective comparison. *J Cataract Refract Surg.* 2010;36(11):1925-1933.

SUGGESTED READING

Shah DN, Melki S. Complications of femtosecond-assisted laser in-situ keratomileusis flaps. *Semin Ophthalmol.* 2014;29(5-6):363-375.

Please see videos on the accompanying website at

www.healio.com/books/lasikvideos

Fifth

12

Decentered Flaps

ETIOLOGY AND INCIDENCE OF DECENTERED FLAPS

Appropriate flap centration is crucial for the success of LASIK. Creating a flap with an adequate diameter is necessary to create a bed that is sufficient for excimer laser treatment. A *decentered flap* is a complication that occurs during the LASIK procedure that can affect the visual and refractive outcome, causing the loss of best-corrected visual acuity if not managed properly. It is important to be prepared to abort the procedure if the exposed stroma cannot accommodate the planned ablation zone.

Patient and surgeon factors can influence flap creation. Head position, ring position, and applanation can all influence the procedure. Decentered flaps have been reported as a complication with mechanical microkeratomes. They mainly occur when the vacuum ring slowly shifts between the application of suction and the initiation of the keratome pass. This is a phenomenon referred to as *oozing;* it can be missed if the surgeon is not attentive to it. Decentered flaps have been reported with less frequency with the femtosecond laser. The femtosecond laser allows small adjustments in flap centration prior to ablation to permit the realignment of the flap. This is not possible with a microkeratome laser. The incidence of decentered flaps after microkeratome LASIK has been reported to be approximately

Melki SA, Fadlallah A.
LASIK Emergencies: A Video Primer (pp 141-146).
© 2018 SLACK Incorporated.

0.6%.[1-3] Only one study in the literature reports the rate of decentration with femtosecond LASIK at approximately 0.1%.[2-4]

FEMTOSECOND LASIK COMPLICATIONS AND IMMEDIATE SOLUTIONS

Complication #1: Difficult Docking Resulting in Decentered Flap

Video section: 0 minutes 10 seconds

Platform: WaveLight FS200 (Alcon Labs)

Flap diameter: 9.3 mm

Flap target depth: 110 microns (μm)

The initial surgery resulted in a decentered flap (video 12; time: 0 minutes 10 seconds; Figures 12-1, 12-2, and 12-3).

Some practical measures are as follows:

- Assess the available stroma for excimer laser treatment.
- Abort the procedure in cases of severely decentered flaps (ie, situation where a 6.0-mm stromal ablation zone is not attainable under the flap).
- Plan for a future surface refractive procedure.

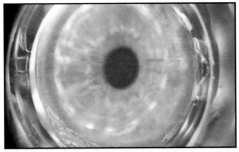

Figure 12-1. Initial surgery showed a difficult docking attempt.

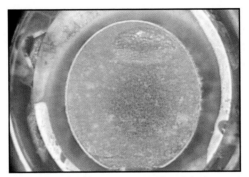

Figure 12-2. Docking was repeated, and the laser cut resulted in an inferiorly decentered flap.

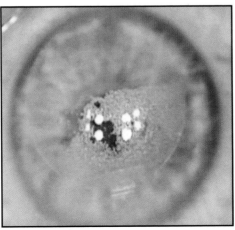

Figure 12-3. Flap was not lifted. A surface refractive procedure was performed 1 week later.

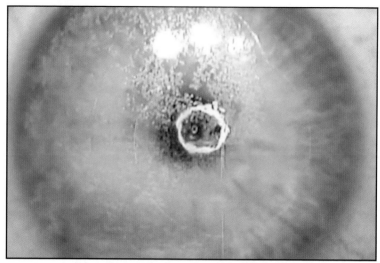

Figure 12-4. Initial surgery resulted in a decentered flap. The flap was repositioned, and the surgery was aborted. A surface refractive procedure was performed 1 week later. At 2 months postoperatively, the flap was clear and well-centered with no signs of epithelial ingrowth. The uncorrected visual acuity was 20/20.

Complication #2: Decentered Thin Irregular Flap

Video section: 1 minute 30 seconds

Platform: IntraLase FS60 kilohertz (kHz) (Abbott Medical Optics)

Flap diameter: 9.3 mm

Flap target depth: 110 μm

The initial surgery resulted in a decentered flap (video 12; time: 1 minute 30 seconds; Figure 12-4).

Some practical measures are as follows:

- Assess the flap regularity and available stroma for excimer laser treatment.
- Abort the procedure when dealing with an irregular flap.
- Place a contact lens.
- Plan for a future refractive procedure.

General Practical Measures in Femtosecond LASIK Surgery

Once decentered flap is detected, the following should occur:

- Assess the flap regularity and available stroma for excimer laser treatment. It is preferable to make that assessment prior to flap lifting.
- Consider shrinking the optical zone if needed. This may be difficult to do if the patient has a large pupil.
- Abort the procedure in cases of severely decentered flaps (ie, situations where the stromal ablation zone is not adequate).
- Abort the procedure if the flap is too irregular to be lifted.
- On occasion, the blend zone may extend beyond the exposed stroma and ablate the surrounding epithelium. This may increase the risk of epithelial ingrowth. A microsponge can be placed on the epithelium to protect it from the overlying excimer ablation.
- Place a contact lens if needed.
- Plan for a future refractive procedure.

PREVENTION OF DECENTERED FLAPS

Femtosecond LASIK

Decentered flaps are usually due to difficult docking. Ensuring adequate suction and minimizing patient factors such as eye movement or squeezing can help to prevent this complication when using femtosecond lasers.

Microkeratome LASIK

The incidence of decentered flaps may be reduced when using microkeratome if the surgeon ensures adequate suction, inspects the blades, adjusts the plate thickness according to corneal curvature, and avoids cutting the flap if the intraocular pressure is low.

REFERENCES

1. Melki SA, Azar DT. LASIK complications: etiology, management, and prevention. *Surv Ophthalmol.* 2001;46(2):95-116.
2. Ang M, Mehta JS, Rosman M, et al. Visual outcomes comparison of 2 femtosecond laser platforms for laser in situ keratomileusis. *J Cataract Refract Surg.* 2013;39(11):1647-1652.
3. Moshirfar M, Gardiner JP, Schliesser J, et al. Laser in situ keratomileusis flap complications using mechanical microkeratome versus femtosecond laser: retrospective comparison. *J Cataract Refract Surg.* 2010;36(11):1925-1933.
4. Shah DN, Melki S. Complications of femtosecond-assisted laser in-situ keratomileusis flaps. *Semin Ophthalmol.* 2014;29(5-6):363-375.

Please see videos on the accompanying website at

www.healio.com/books/lasikvideos

13

Subconjunctival Hemorrhage and Bleeding

ETIOLOGY AND INCIDENCE OF SUBCONJUNCTIVAL HEMORRHAGE AND BLEEDING

Femtosecond LASIK

Subconjunctival hemorrhage can occur with IntraLase platforms (Abbott Medical Optics) when the syringe is applied too quickly or released too quickly during the suction application. It can also occur when multiple suction applications are needed due to suction loss. Bleeding from limbal vessels may also occur at the edge of the flap. It is seen most commonly in patients with limbal neovascularization and prior contact lens use. Limbal neovascularization as a result of rosacea, atopy, and meibomian gland dysfunction may also contribute to subconjunctival hemorrhage. Subconjunctival hemorrhage incidence is noted in 68.9% of eyes with the IntraLase (Abbott Medical Optics) platform but none with the VisuMax Femtosecond Laser (Zeiss).[1] This is thought to be secondary to the variation in the docking mechanisms. For instance, suction is applied to the sclera with the IntraLase laser as compared to cornea with the VisuMax laser.[1] Bleeding incidence is less than 1% with the femtosecond laser.

Melki SA, Fadlallah A.
LASIK Emergencies: A Video Primer (pp 147-154).
© 2018 SLACK Incorporated.

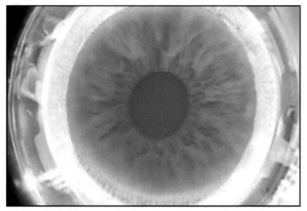

Figure 13-1. Photograph showing a large peripheral flap and peripheral vessels transected.

Microkeratome LASIK

Subconjunctival hemorrhage can occur with microkeratome LASIK from the suction ring. Micropannus formation is commonly seen with soft contact lens wear, and hemorrhage may occur if the microkeratome pass transects these vessels. This complication may be frequently encountered with larger flaps (9 to 9.5 mm) and larger treatment zones needed for hyperopia. With the microkeratome, subconjunctival hemorrhage incidence is between 50% and 70%.[3] Bleeding incidence is less than 1% with the microkeratome.[1,3]

FEMTOSECOND LASIK COMPLICATIONS AND IMMEDIATE SOLUTIONS

Complication #1: Large Peripheral Flap

Video section: 0 minutes 5 seconds
Platform: WaveLight FS200 (Alcon Labs)
Flap diameter: 9.5 mm
Flap target depth: 110 microns (µm)

The initial surgery resulted in subconjunctival hemorrhage and bleeding in the interface (video 13; time: 0 minutes 5 seconds; Figures 13-1, 13-2, 13-3, and 13-4).

Some practical measures are as follows:

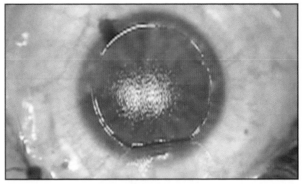

Figure 13-2. Photograph showing blood reaching the stromal bed.

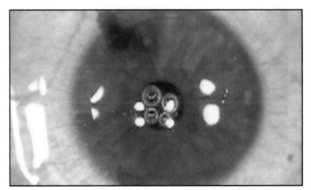

Figure 13-3. Dry the stromal interface before applying the excimer laser.

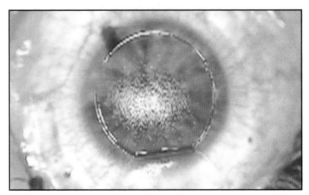

Figure 13-4. Irrigate the interface after treatment to avoid any residual blood.

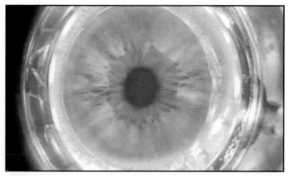

Figure 13-5. Photograph showing difficult docking.

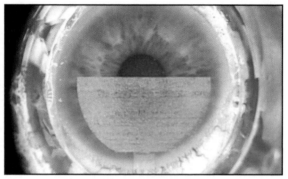

Figure 13-6. Photograph showing scleral show and peripheral blood vessels transected.

- Dry the blood from the interface before applying excimer laser treatment.
- Keep drying the periphery during laser treatment.
- Irrigate the interface to avoid any residual blood.

Complication #2: Several Docking Attempts

Video section: 2 minutes 0 seconds

Platform: WaveLight FS200

Flap diameter: 9.3 mm

Flap target depth: 110 μm

The initial surgery on the left eye resulted in subconjunctival hemorrhage and bleeding from the hinge zone after several difficult docking attempts (video 13; time: 2 minutes 0 seconds; Figures 13-5, 13-6, 13-7, and 13-8).

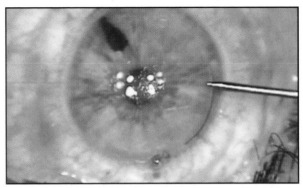

Figure 13-7. Photograph showing the bleeding of vessels near the hinge area.

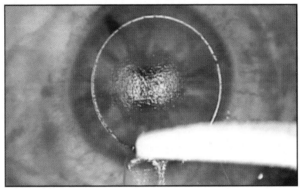

Figure 13-8. Dry the stromal interface before applying the treatment. Excimer laser treatment (WaveLight EX500 [Alcon Labs]) was then uneventful. Irrigating the interface after treatment was also performed to avoid any blood in the interface.

Some practical measures are as follows:
- Dry the interface before applying excimer laser treatment.
- Keep drying the periphery during laser treatment.
- Irrigate the interface to avoid any residual blood.

General Practical Measures in Femtosecond LASIK Surgery

Once subconjunctival hemorrhage is detected, the following should occur:

- Continue the laser treatment.
- Exert downward pressure with a sponge to stop any active conjunctival bleeding.
- Dry well before and during the laser treatment to avoid irregular astigmatism.
- Irrigate any blood from the interface after the laser treatment to decrease the risk of diffuse lamellar keratitis.

Even though a subconjunctival hemorrhage is generally of no consequence, it is important to inform patients of the risk so that they are not alarmed.

Microkeratome LASIK Complications and Immediate Solutions

Complication #3: Large Peripheral Flap

Video section: 4 minutes 24 seconds
Platform: Hansatome (Bausch + Lomb)
Flap diameter: 9.5 mm
Flap target depth: 120 μm

The initial surgery resulted in bleeding (video 13; time: 4 minutes 24 seconds; Figure 13-9).

Some practical measures are as follows:

- Dry the interface before applying excimer laser treatment.
- Keep drying the periphery during laser treatment.
- Irrigate the interface to avoid any residual blood.

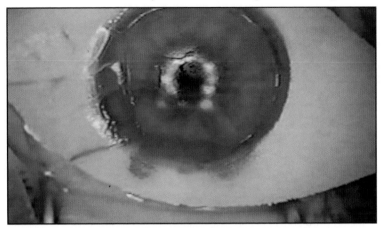

Figure 13-9. Dry the stromal interface before applying the treatment.

General Practical Measures in Microkeratome LASIK Surgery

Once subconjunctival hemorrhage is detected, the following should occur:

- Exert downward pressure with a sponge to stop any active conjunctival bleeding.
- Dry well before and during the laser treatment to avoid irregular astigmatism.
- Irrigate any blood from the interface after the laser treatment to decrease the risk of diffuse lamellar keratitis.
- If associated with an irregular flap, the surgery should be aborted.

Even though a subconjunctival hemorrhage is generally of no consequence, it is important to inform patients of the risk so that they are not alarmed.

PREVENTION OF SUBCONJUNCTIVAL HEMORRHAGE AND BLEEDING

The slow and controlled application of suction and release is important in preventing bleeding. Large peripheral flaps are more commonly associated with an increased risk of transecting peripheral blood vessels. Flaps that are decentered and closer to the limbus on one side are also at greater risk. Avoiding superior flap decentration and making a smaller flap can prevent bleeding in patients with neovascularization. Although brimonidine has been used in the past to minimize the risk of bleeding, it has been reported to increase the risk of flap dislocation.[2]

REFERENCES

1. Rosman M, Hall RC, Chan C, et al. Comparison of efficacy and safety of laser in situ keratomileusis using 2 femtosecond laser platforms in contralateral eyes. *J Cataract Refract Surg.* 2013;39(7):1066-1073.
2. Aslanides IM, Tsiklis NS, Ozkilic E, Coskunseven E, Pallikaris IG, Jankov MR. The effect of topical apraclonidine on subconjunctival hemorrhage and flap adherence in LASIK patients. *J Refract Surg.* 2006;22(6):585-588.
3. Yildirim R, Devranoglu K, Ozdamar A, Aras C, Ozkiris A, Ozkan S. Flap complications in our learning curve of laser in situ keratomileusis using the Hansatome microkeratome. *Eur J Ophthalmol.* 2001;11(4):328-332.

SUGGESTED READING

Feder R, Rapuano C. *The LASIK Handbook: A Case-Based Approach.* Second edition. Philadelphia, PA: Lippincott Williams & Wilkins; 2013.
Shah DN, Melki S. Complications of femtosecond-assisted laser in-situ keratomileusis flaps. *Semin Ophthalmol.* 2014;29(5-6):363-375.

Please see videos on the accompanying website at

www.healio.com/books/lasikvideos

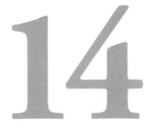

Special Considerations

DIFFICULT DOCKING

The following are 5 main factors that may coexist and result in difficult docking: small palpebral fissure (Figure 14-1), lid squeezing, conjunctival chalasis (Figure 14-2), deep orbit, and particular nose shape.

Small Palpebral Fissure

In patients with narrow palpebral fissures, space is limited. Turning an individual's head away from the eye that is having surgery causes the eyeball to rotate away from the nose, and creates extra space to place the suction ring. A lid speculum may be used to give better exposure to get the vacuum ring onto the globe.

Lid Squeezing

This may exert pressure on the suction ring, and lead to loss of suction. Prompting the patient to relax and adding an anesthetic drop may help. Furthermore, putting an anesthetic in the fellow eye and asking the patient to keep that eye open can assist in keeping the surgical eye open. Using a lid speculum may improve exposure to get the vacuum ring into the eye and counteract lid squeezing.

Melki SA, Fadlallah A.
LASIK Emergencies: A Video Primer (pp 155-159).
© 2018 SLACK Incorporated.

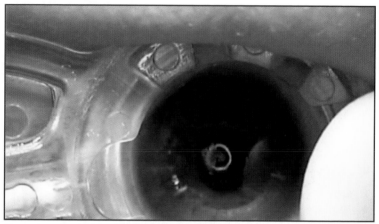

Figure 14-1. Docking with a small palpebral fissure.

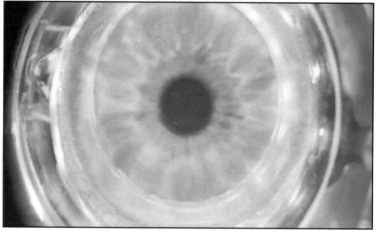

Figure 14-2. Photograph showing conjunctival chalasis and lid squeezing during a docking attempt.

Conjunctival Chalasis

Sometimes, patients have loose redundant conjunctiva. In these cases, the conjunctiva closes the suction port rather than the eyeball itself, giving pseudosuction. Pushing the lid speculum down (if used during docking) or pushing the conjunctiva away with a suction ring (prior to suction initiation) may help to initiate suction.

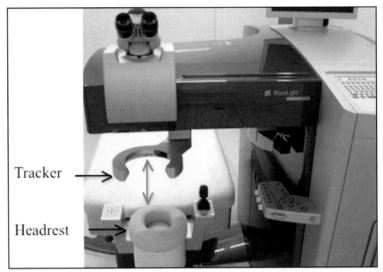

Figure 14-3. Relationship between the tracking system and the headrest.

Deep Orbit

In patients with deep orbit, docking is more difficult due to difficult access to the surface of the eye. Pushing down slightly on the lid speculum (if used during docking) can help to get more clearance. Using a lid speculum may improve exposure to get the vacuum ring onto the globe.

Particular Nose Shape

A large nose can make docking more difficult. With femtosecond LASIK, the applanation cone can become hindered by the nose during docking. With microkeratome LASIK, the microkeratome head may become hindered by the nose during rotation or a translation movement. Turning the patient's head away from the eye that is having surgery causes the eyeball to rotate away from the nose and therefore improves exposure.

CHEST CONFIGURATION INTERFERING WITH TRACKER

Some excimer platforms (eg WaveLight EX500 [Alcon Labs]) use an eye tracker system that moves downward toward the eye upon activation (Figure 14-3). This requires a free space between the tracking system and the upper part of the chest. In some cases (eg, obesity, macromastia, kyphotic neck or spine), this space is reduced and the tracker hits the chest and deactivates.

Some practical measures are as follows:

- Move the headrest upward: This allows the bed to move downward to focus the laser on the surface of the eye. Moving the bed down increases the space between the tracking system and the upper part of the chest.
- Ask the assistant to press on the upper part of the patient's chest down and toward the feet: This may create some space between the tracking system and the upper part of the chest.

ANXIOUS PATIENT

One of the most common fears about LASIK surgery is pain. Many prospective LASIK patients are afraid that they will experience discomfort since the procedure is performed while they are fully conscious. A mild sedative (eg, diazepam 10 mg) is given to patients to ensure that they remain comfortable during the procedure, and numbing drops are applied to the eyes before the surgery begins.

Relaxation techniques can also work.[1] The following types of relaxation techniques exist: autogenic relaxation, progressive muscle relaxation, and visualization. With autogenic relaxation, visual imagery and body awareness are used to reduce stress. A person repeats words or suggestions in his or her mind to relax, both mentally and physically. With progressive muscle relaxation, a patient focuses on the difference between muscle tension and relaxation to become more aware of physical sensation. This is done by tensing muscles for 5 seconds and relaxing them for 30 seconds. A good place to start would be the toes. Visualization involves forming mental images of calming places or situations. The object is, not just to visualize, but also to use as many senses as possible, including smell, sight, sound, and touch.

On rare occasions, one will encounter patients who have extreme anxiety—if not an outright phobia—about an eye examination. Not only will they refuse all drops, but there is also absolute defiance toward any tonometry or touching of the eyelids. If feasible, these cases can be done under general anesthesia in a surgery center.

REFERENCE

1. Kamath PS. A novel distraction technique for pain management during local anesthesia administration in pediatric patients. *J Clin Pediatr Dent.* 2013;38(1):45-47.

SUGGESTED READING

Shah DN, Melki S. Complications of femtosecond-assisted laser in-situ keratomileusis flaps. *Semin Ophthalmol.* 2014;29(5-6):363-375.

Syed ZA, Melki SA. Successful femtosecond LASIK flap creation despite multiple suction losses. *Digit J Ophthalmol.* 2014;20(1):7-9.

15

Management of Postoperative Complications

VISION REHABILITATION FOR CORNEAS WITH BUTTONHOLE

A buttonholed flap occurs when the microkeratome blade travels more superficially than intended and enters the epithelium/Bowman's complex. Buttonholes may be partial thickness if they transect the Bowman's layer or full thickness if they exit through the epithelium. The incidence of buttonholes ranges between 0.2% and 0.56%.[1] This is the most common complication in microkeratome LASIK, resulting in the loss of best-corrected visual acuity (BCVA). Risk factors include the following:

- High keratometric values.
- Previous incisional keratotomy.
- Pre-existing surface lesion (eg, pterygiums, corneal scars).

Management

While some recommend proceeding with scraping the epithelium and performing a photorefractive keratectomy (PRK)/LASIK laser ablation (Figures 15-1 and 15-2), this approach may not be feasible in high myopic patients due to the appearance of subepithelial haze.

Melki SA, Fadlallah A.
LASIK Emergencies: A Video Primer (pp 161-171).
© 2018 SLACK Incorporated.

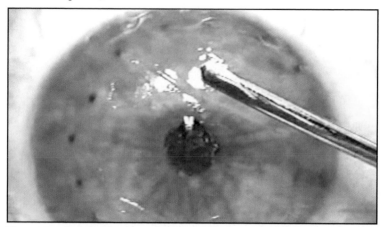

Figure 15-1. Epithelial flap lifting after alcohol application for 40s.

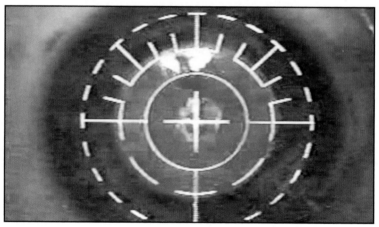

Figure 15-2. Successful excimer laser treatment. At the patient's 2-month follow-up visit, his uncorrected distance visual acuity was 20/20. No epithelial ingrowth was observed.

Using a no-touch transepithelial PRK within 2 weeks may prevent irregular astigmatism formation from the uneven ablation profile resulting from any late scar formation.

Video: 0 minutes 5 seconds; LASIK 3 months over buttonhole.

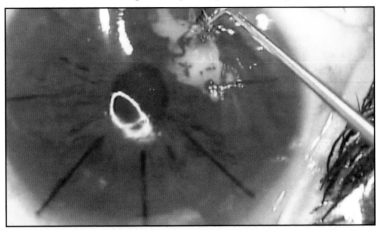

Figure 15-3. Identifying and lifting the flap edge carefully to avoid flap tear due to underlying scarring or melting.

EPITHELIAL INGROWTH

Implantation of epithelial cells in the interface may be due to seeding during surgery or migration under the flap. Most of these cells will disappear without consequences. More concerning is epithelial ingrowth that is contiguous with the flap edge. This can progress to involve the visual axis with irregular astigmatism and possible flap melting. Epithelial growth at the interface may be more common after enhancement procedures due to adjacent epithelial abrasions with increased cell proliferation.

Management

Nonprogressive epithelial ingrowth should be monitored. Hyperopic shift is an early indicator of possible underlying stromal melt. This may result in loss of BCVA. Epithelial cells under the LASIK flap should be managed aggressively if they progress toward the visual axis or if they induce stromal melting. The flap is lifted, the stromal bed and the flap undersurface are thoroughly irrigated and scraped, and the flap is repositioned (Figures 15-3, 15-4, 15-5, and 15-6). Epithelial cell debridement can be achieved mechanically with a #15 blade or with dedicated instruments (eg, Yaghouti LASIK Polisher [ASICO]), or by using excimer laser bursts in phototherapeutic keratectomy mode.

Video: 0 minutes 58 seconds

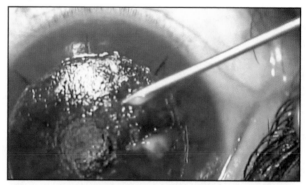

Figure 15-4. Scrape the bed with a blade and/or a LASIK flap lifter.

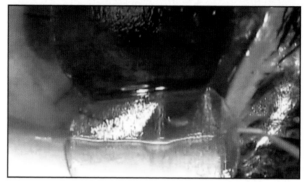

Figure 15-5. Scrape the flap. A closed speculum can be used as a working platform by asking the patient to look superiorly.

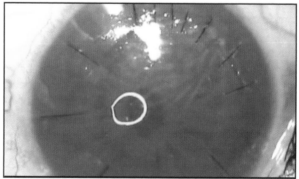

Figure 15-6. Flap suturing at the area of epithelial ingrowth to decrease the risk of cell migration under the flap.

FLAP FOLDS AND STRIAE

Striae and folds are both seen commonly after LASIK and can be visually symptomatic. Causes have been hypothesized to include mechanical disruption; dryness of the flap leading to shrinkage; misalignment; and changes in the corneal contour, specifically in high myopic correction. If they involve the visual axis, folds can induce irregular astigmatism and the loss of BCVA. Striae are rare, with an incidence that varies between 1% and 2.4%.[2]

Management

Management can range from light stroking with a moist microsponge or instrument at the slit lamp to lifting the flap and stretching radially followed by repositioning (Figures 15-7, 15-8, and 15-9). Recalcitrant folds may require the removal of the central epithelium as it may prevent the flattening of the folds due to epithelial hyperplasia in the crevices formed by the folds. Suturing the flap can also be considered if the striae do not resolve (Figure 15-10). Flap folds are managed more successfully if the intervention is initiated as soon as they are recognized to be visually significant.

Video: 3 minutes 45 seconds

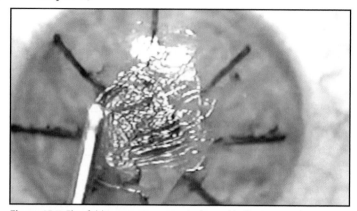

Figure 15-7. Flap folds are more apparent after epithelium removal.

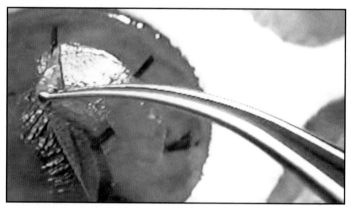

Figure 15-8. Lift the flap gently to avoid flap tears.

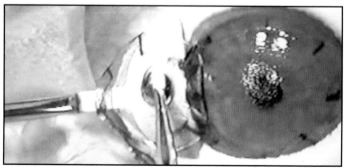

Figure 15-9. Stretch the flap radially, and massage the underside of the flap.

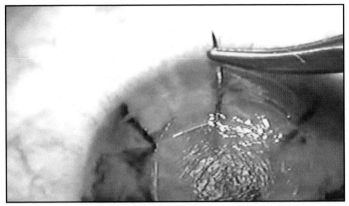

Figure 15-10. Flap suturing at 2 opposite positions allows the stretching of the flap and results in striae resolution.

FLAP TRAUMA AND DISLOCATION

Dislocated flaps can occur any time after surgery and most commonly present with acute pain and a decrease in vision. Etiology often includes mechanical trauma to the flap. In the early postoperative period (first 24 hours), they can be secondary to minor manipulations such as rubbing the eye or squeezing following the procedure. More significant trauma is needed to dislocate the flap afterwards. Flap dislocations 1 day following LASIK vary between 1.1% in femtosecond LASIK and 2.5% in microkeratome LASIK.[1,2]

Management

A dislodged flap should be repositioned immediately (Figures 15-11 and 15-12). Generally, the longer it has been since the displacement, the more extensive the treatment, as epithelial hyperplasia may fill the crevices of the folded flap. The underside of the flap and the stromal bed may need to be scraped to remove any epithelial ingrowth. Any folds should be stretched out, and epithelial debridement may be needed to flatten any recalcitrant flap folds.

Video: 6 minutes 32 seconds

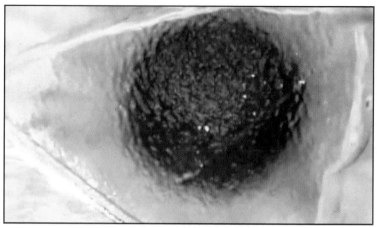

Figure 15-11. Localized flap trauma. Clean the bed, irrigate the interface, and then reposition the flap.

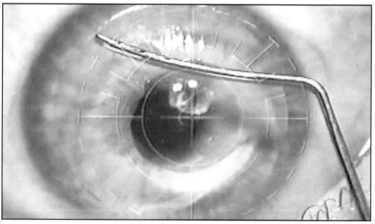

Figure 15-12. Photograph showing post-traumatic flap dislocation, bed irrigation, and flap repositioning.

PERSISTENT EPITHELIAL DEFECT

Concern involves large epithelial defects, especially those with a connection to the flap edge. The incidence of epithelial defects with LASIK was reported to be approximately 5%.[1,2] The proliferating epithelial cells might migrate under the flap edge. Associated inflammation can also lead to the

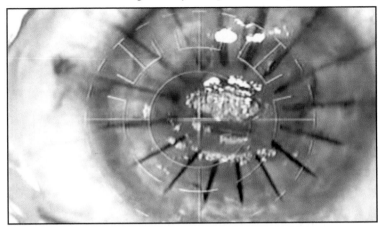

Figure 15-13. Persistent epithelial defect on a LASIK flap.

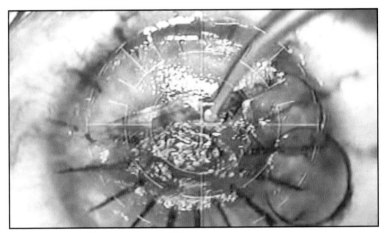

Figure 15-14. Lift flap gently to avoid flap tears.

melting of the surrounding flap tissue. Increased risk of diffuse lamellar keratitis in patients with epithelial defects has also been observed.

Management

If an epithelial defect is noted intraoperatively, a higher index of suspicion for epithelial ingrowth should be maintained (Figures 15-13, 15-14, 15-15, and 15-16). An attempt at repositioning the loose epithelium should be performed. Alternatively, the epithelium can be gently debrided and a contact lens can be applied. These measures help with pain control and with

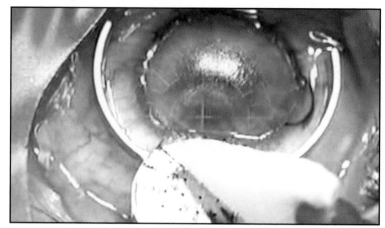

Figure 15-15. Scrape flap. A Melki LASIK flap stabilizer (Rhein Medical, Inc) can be used for this step.

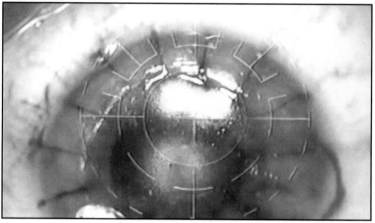

Figure 15-16. Flap suturing at 2 opposite positions may help to keep the flap edge flattened, allowing an easier path for epithelial cells to repopulate the flap surface.

improving flap adherence and preventing epithelial cell ingrowth. Topical nonsteroidal anti-inflammatory drugs may also be useful to ease the associated discomfort, but they may be associated with the induction of sterile infiltrates.

Video: 8 minutes 44 seconds

REFERENCES

1. Melki SA, Azar DT. LASIK complications: etiology, management, and prevention. *Surv Ophthalmol.* 2001;46(2):95-116.
2. Shah DN, Melki S. Complications of femtosecond-assisted laser in-situ keratomileusis flaps. *Semin Ophthalmol.* 2014;29(5-6):363-375.

Please see videos on the accompanying website at

www.healio.com/books/lasikvideos

Index